W9-APM-368

The Fungus Link

The Fungus Link

An Introduction to
Fungal Disease

Including the Initial Phase Diet

Doug A. Kaufmann

edited by

Beverly Thornhill Hunt, Ph.D.

MediaTrition
Rockwall, Texas

Copyright © 2000 by Doug A. Kaufmann
All rights reserved.

Second edition produced by Chris Nygaard
(intexdfw@yahoo.com)

Published by MediaTrition, Inc.
301 W. Washington Street
Rockwall, Texas 75087
(972)772-0990

All material is for informational purposes only. This book is a compiled report of existing data and research and does not take the place of professional advice from your health care provider. The authors and publisher assume no responsibility concerning the use of information herein. Approaches described within this book are not offered as cures, prescriptions, or diagnoses. As always, consult your doctor before beginning any new treatment.

Publisher's Cataloging-in-Publication
(provided by Quality Books, Inc.)

Kaufmann, Doug A., 1949-
    The fungus link : an introduction to fungal
disease,
    including the initial phase diet / by Doug A.
Kaufmann ;
    edited by Beverly Thornhill Hunt. – 1st ed.
    p. cm.
    Includes bibliographical references and index.
    ISBN: 0-9703418-0-6

    1. Mycoses – Popular works. 2. Medical
mycology –
    Popular works. 3. Pathogenic fungi.   I. Title

Manufactured in the United States of America

First Edition of The Fungus Link edited by Beverly Thornhill Hunt. Cover design of both editions by Christine Hunt.

Introduction
to the Revised Edition

Much has changed since Doug Kaufmann — with the help of Dr. David Holland and a number of other, health care professionals — published the original *Fungus Link*. Doug's nationally broadcast TV show, *Your Health*, continues to grow in popularity. Dr. Dave is now a fully-licensed, family practice physician. He and Doug spend most weekends conducting health seminars in cities all over the United States. In place of the *Fungazette* newsletter from which *The Fungus Link* was compiled, the two have launched a health care website by the name of "iknowthecause.com." Please have a look.

Regarding content, a few, selected elements have been revised and updated for this, the second edition. Typography, layout and structure have been reworked. We have also added a week's worth of sample menus for the *Initial Phase Diet* (formerly known as the *Phase 1 Diet*) and *Your Fungal Quotient*, a questionnaire to aid you in determining whether fungi might lie behind your health problems.

Mediatrition has recently added three titles to its list: *The Germ that Causes Cancer*, *Infectious Diabetes* and *The Fungus Link, Volume 2*. For information on these, or to order, please click on the website or call (972)772-0990.

-Chris Nygaard

Foreword

I have known Doug Kaufmann for many years, have had many patients in common with him, and have come to respect his work as a nutritionist and as a fungal expert. In this book, you will read practical information about what fungal illness is, how common a health problem it is, how to recognize it by its symptoms, and how to eradicate it from the body. The testimonials presented give strong support to the seriousness and frequency of fungal illness as a human health problem. I, too, have seen in my own practice fungi representing the primary underlying cause of diverse health conditions including chronic fatigue syndrome, crippling arthritis, severe intestinal disorders, chronic allergies, chronic respiratory illness, "brain fog" syndrome, depression, and chronic skin conditions (eczema, psoriasis, pruritic dermatitis). The sections written by other health professionals prove that fungal illness is being recognized by more and more doctors for its serious impact on human health.

If you or someone you love has a chronic illness, read this book thoroughly. Next, reflect on or pray about what you have read. Then strongly consider changing your diet (or the diet of your loved one) for a few weeks to starve the fungi (as described in the appendix). Even consider taking some anti-fungal herbals (also described in the appendix) or prescription anti-fungal medications if you can find a doctor who will assist you. When you do these things and you initially feel worse (described in this book as the Herxheimer "die off" reaction) then days later feel better than you have in a long time, you probably had fungi causing much of your illness. Become proactive, take charge of your own health, and seek out a health practitioner who understands the effect of fungal illness and related conditions on your health. Read, learn, implement what you learn, and be well!

Wm. Lee Cowden, M. D.

co-author: <u>*Alternative Medicine*</u>
<u>*Definitive Guide to Cancer*</u> and
<u>*Cancer Diagnosis: What To Do Next*</u>

Preface

In 1996, Dr. David Holland and I were busy gathering data to confirm our suspicions that what we had been observing clinically had scientific validity. For the previous 25 years, I had been able to assist people with many diseases and symptoms by addressing a germ that physicians had completely missed in their diagnoses. There are today approximately 80 documented autoimmune diseases, each one without an etiological basis (known cause). Scientists have no idea what causes the heart attacks and cancers that kill one million people annually. In medicine, the word "germ" is often used synonymously with the word "bacteria." This, in a small way, illustrates the confusion regarding the causes of disease among even the brightest medical practitioners and scientists.

So it is that the first book we know of to implicate fungus as the cause of debilitation and death has been completed. As you peruse these pages, know that this work includes scientific notation and confirmation of the hypothesis that disease *does* have a known pathogen and is *not* bacterial in every instance!

I suppose the invention of antibiotics was viewed as revolutionary by those in 1950s science. Our brightest, best scientists concluded that we had finally defeated the germs responsible for causing sickness and disease. If this were true, 1955 should have been a banner year in science. Certainly those millions who took antibiotics in that five year time span were now less vulnerable to common maladies. If not, they reasoned, then perhaps more antibiotics would permanently fix them. I have often used the analogy of calcium intake and osteoporosis in America to prove my point before surrendering to the notion that antibiotics were not the magic bullet hoped for. If osteoporosis were due to calcium deficiency, Americans would never have osteoporosis. Today, celebrity white moustaches abound, beckoning us to drink more milk! Between the calcium supplements we throw down our throats and the amount of milk that we drink, our bones should never become fragile!

Yet the opposite is true in each of these situations. Osteoporosis is striking more Americans than ever before in history, despite dairy intake and calcium supplementation. Bacteria continue to elude even the best antibiotics, despite the billions of dollars of pharmaceutical research. Unless the etiology (cause) of a disease is identified, all the supplements and drugs in the world may be for naught.

Early in the year 2000, researchers discovered that the density of the bones of laboratory mice improved up to 50 percent when they were given cholesterol-lowering drugs. It is even more important to note that cholesterol-lowering drugs are antifungal medications. That brings us full circle.

This book is a compilation of data originally published from 1997 to 1999 in our newsletter, *The Fungazette*. The Fungus Link is designed to help our readers locate the possible cause of their health maladies. It seems an especially lonely existence when you are sick and no one knows why. This book does not replace the diagnosis, prognosis, or treatment that your health care practitioner can provide. But it is my hope that, in time, the competency at diagnosing fungal disease will improve. I can assure you that will happen if medical protocol will call for proper diet and antifungal herbs or medicines for their difficult patients. There is nothing more convincing than observing life threatening diseases frequently respond favorably to simple antifungal therapy.

This book is dedicated to...

...the living and deceased patients
erroneously diagnosed
with a serious disease
when all the while
they were actually suffering
from an undiagnosed,
fungal condition

...and the open-minded physicians
who help the sick and prevent
pain, suffering and death
by treating every symptom and disease
for which we do not know the cause
as though it were induced by fungi.

Your peers will scoff, but
your patients will flourish.

Table of Contents

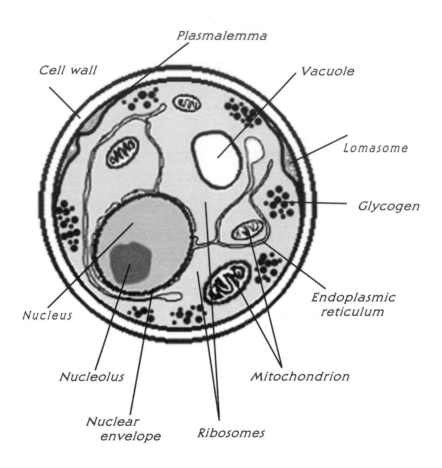

Cell wall

Plasmalemma

Vacuole

Lomasome

Glycogen

Endoplasmic
reticulum

Nucleus

Nucleolus

Mitochondrion

Nuclear
envelope

Ribosomes

Cross section of a generalized fungus cell

FUNGUS

A simple plant
that lacks chlorophyll.
Fungi include the yeasts, rust,
molds and mushrooms.
They live as either
saprophytes or parasites
of plants and animals (man).
Some species infect
and cause disease in man.

- The Bantam Medical Dictionary

Chapter One

Fungi and Your Health

A doctor's introduction to nutrition and fungus

Roby Mitchell, Ph.D., M.D.

Greetings to all of you! I want to congratulate you for taking the time to educate yourself on being an active participant in improving your health. You are, potentially, the best doctor you could ever have.

I'd like to begin by introducing myself to you and letting you know how Doug and I became associated. My background is in traditional western medicine. I graduated with honors from Texas Tech School of Medicine. Subsequently, I started a practice as an emergency room physician. The emergency room is the epitome of acute care medicine, so I saw lots of patients suffering from symptoms of diseases that had not been adequately addressed for years. Many fell under the category of vascular disease, which includes "heart attack" and stroke. These problems develop after years of investing in lifestyle choices that clog up the arteries of the heart and brain.

What made me begin to question the way I practiced medicine was the number of young people, 45 to 60, that came in to the emergency room with these problems. It is traumatic to go out into the waiting room and tell a family that their loved one is dead, but it is heartrending when it is a relatively young mother and her children who have just lost their husband, father, and breadwinner.

Reading the medical literature of the time also engendered some discomfort, as it was reporting that upwards of 80% of these tragic events were completely preventable by implementing some relatively simple lifestyle changes. I was telling that young mother and her children that "we did all that we could do," but obviously that was not the case.

During my medical school training, I was chosen to participate in a student exchange program between Texas Tech and Jinan University in Canton, China. There I studied Chinese traditional medicine, which included the use of foods, herbal medicines, and acupuncture to treat disease. Their philosophy focused on getting the whole body system back into balance and allowing the body's intelligence to do the healing. The physician was an assistant or facilitator. I was starting to wonder if this was not a more appropriate way to reestablish health.

Coincidental with these ruminations was the release of a study done by Dr. Dean Ornish. He had proven that you could open up clogged arteries by implementing a regime of exercise, stress reduction, and healthful eating. This could save millions in health care costs each year and prevent patients from undergoing the risks and trauma of surgical procedures.

Seeing more and more MDs start to adopt this philosophy, I started a little sideline practice that focused on teaching patients lifestyle changes instead of always relying on medications. Once the word got out that there was an M.D. in Amarillo, Texas, who focused on natural healing, my phone started ringing off the wall. I found myself spending more time in this type of practice, even though I also continued my E.R. practice. This led to my doing a self-study course on nutrition and its link to disease. I learned how nutrients from plant sources were being used to prevent and treat many diseases.

During my investigations, I ran across a product called Juice Plus that was being touted as being the alternative to juicing. I had never taken supplements in the past, but I knew that I was not getting the recommended amount of raw fruits and vegetables in my diet. I was so impressed after having this product analyzed that I started taking it. Within two to three weeks, I felt increased energy, improved quality of sleep, improved regularity, and my recovery time after workouts decreased (I participate in triathlons). I had similarly impressive results with my mom, dad, and other family members. It wasn't long before I, who had been staunchly anti-vitamin mineral supplementation, was being asked to speak across the United States, Canada, and Europe on the benefits of these whole food capsules that replaced juicing several pounds of organic fruits and organic vegetables.

One of the places I was asked to speak was on a then little-known health talk show hosted by who else? Doug Kaufmann. Doug and I became fast friends as we shared similar convictions about the role of individual responsibility in health care and the benefits of nutritional supplements in preventing and treating diseases. I also found Doug to share a similar skepticism and integrity.

Fortunately for me, Doug became not only a friend but also a mentor. I'm relatively new at practicing the type of medicine that Doug has been espousing and training other medical professionals in for over 20 years. So far, the most important lesson he has taught me is the association of a wide variety of clinical syndromes with systemic (all over the body) candidiasis, commonly known as yeast.

This has been a much-maligned diagnosis in the past because it has eluded laboratory verification. However, because of the scientific verification Doug presented to me, as well as the trust I had developed in his clinical expertise, I started treating patients who fit the yeast profile. A combination of prescriptive antifungals, a diet devoid of refined sugars and yeasts, immune system enhancement via supplements, and replacement of "good" intestinal bacteria genuinely helped these patients.

The results have been nothing short of miraculous for many patients. Many had suffered for years with symptoms of chronic fatigue, PMS, depression, irritable bowel, obesity, attention deficit disorder, asthma, interstitial cystitis, bladder incontinence, prostatitis, psoriasis, MS, and fibromyalgia. They dramatically improved if they followed the treatment protocol.

I can't thank Doug enough for teaching me about this life-changing therapy. My patients would thank him, too, if they knew that he was responsible for teaching me. However, in order to maintain my status as a near-deity, I've decided to keep that a secret!

-R.M.

What the experts say about fungal diseases

by Doug A. Kaufmann

There is certainly no shortage of scientific literature about fungal symptoms and diseases. And the twentieth century holds nothing as far as knowledge of the many diseases caused by fungus. Just open a Bible and go directly to Leviticus 14 verses 34 and 35. This talk of fungus causing health problems is not new.

As far as twentieth century fungal experts, consider Dr. Lida Mattman, a professor emeritus at Wayne State University. In her excellent book *Stealth Pathogens*, Dr. Mattman asks, "Are fungi in blood smears overlooked because they are confused with blood cells?" She answers a resounding, "Yes!" From that one statement alone, just imagine how many blood conditions are misdiagnosed because machines or laboratory technologists just can't differentiate between spores and cells.

Another bold statement is made on the same page. This one by Dr. M. G. Rinaldi, who says, "Given the right immunocompromised host, virtually any fungus can kill a human being."

29

David Holland, M.D., has a book in his office called *Clinical Mycology* by C. C. Kibbler. (Mycology is the study of fungus.) In this book, published in 1995, 18 prominent physicians from large research universities like Duke, the University of Texas and Stanford expound on the serious health threats that fungi pose. Here are some of the chapters in *Medical Mycology*: Fungal Disease of the Bone and Joint; Fungal Diseases of the Cardiovascular System; Mycoses [fungi] causing mass lesions of the Central Nervous System; Fungal Diseases in Dermatology; Fungal Infections of the Ear, Nose, and Throat; Fungal Infections of the Gastrointestinal Tract; Fungal Infections of the Respiratory Tract; and even Fungal Diseases in Opthalmology. Wouldn't you think every doctor in the world would understand that these microorganisms might cause disease? Why don't they? I am glad you asked!

Most doctors believe that fungus only infects immunocompromised (lowered immunity) patients. If this were true, then San Joaquin Valley Fever, caused by breathing the fungus *Coccidioides immitus*, could not have possibly killed young, healthy military men. What about the ABC episode of *Primetime* aired April 9, 1997, dealing with infants who are sick and dying from fungal exposure in their homes? Or are women who suffer from vaginal yeast infections immuno-compromised? In each of these instances, the integrity of the immune system was only challenged AFTER fungal exposure – not before. So, who is immunocompromised? Are the air we breathe and the water we drink compromising our immune systems? How about the medicines that most Americans take? Since antibiotics are mycotoxins (fungal poisons), perhaps we can now define compromised immunity as applying to anyone who has ever taken an antibiotic! That is certainly a lot of people, but while you ponder that potential statistic, the following may put it in perspective for you.

In 1963, Dr. Harold T. Hyman published in *The Complete Home Medical Encyclopedia* that approximately one-half of the population of the United States had, at one time or another, suffered from a fungal disorder that had been "unrecognized." Now, my question for you is: has medical science really progressed since 1963? Or are 125,000,000 Americans still suffering from "unrecognized" fungal disorders?

Chapter Two

Fungi and Arthritis

Arthritis:
the fungus connection

David Holland, M.D.

The painful fact about most forms of arthritis is that, with the exception of some infectious arthritis conditions, the cause is unknown. For example, the Arthritis Foundation describes rheumatoid arthritis as a "chronic, systemic, inflammatory disorder of unknown etiology."[1] Etiology simply means "the cause or origin" of a disease.

What does fungus have to do with arthritis? First, we'll read what several doctors have to say about the connection, and then we will visit, first hand, the story of one of our patients. Fungi can cause arthritis by either infecting a joint directly, usually spreading via the blood from the primary infection (e.g., the lungs or intestines), or they may indirectly affect a joint by giving off fungal poisons or "mycotoxins." When this happens, several different types of arthritis may occur.

Let's start with gout. Nearly every medical school in the country teaches that gout is caused by uric acid which, when reaching critical levels, forms crystals in the joints. These crystals cause inflammation and are followed by excruciating pain. Dr. A. V.

Costantini, M.D., retired head of the World Health Organization (WHO) Center for Mycotoxins in Food, disagrees. At a 1994 symposium held in Toronto, Canada, Dr. Costantini presented a series of studies by fellow researchers showing that we can't prove that the human body can even manufacture uric acid. In fact, he said, uric acid in the blood stream is more likely of fungal origin.[2] It is the result of fungus entering the body from outside. Furthermore, the studies showed that the urate crystals found in patients with gout occurred days after the inflammation had already set in! Urate crystals were not the cause of the pain experienced by gout patients. So sure was Dr. Costantini of this research that he offered $1,000 to anyone who could prove that the human body created uric acid. As of today, he is not a penny poorer!

Now, let's examine rheumatoid arthritis. In the January 1995 edition of *The Townsend Letter for Doctors*, 19 doctors wrote that a condition known as candidiasis (from the yeast *Candida albicans*) could mimic symptoms associated with rheumatoid arthritis.[3] Dr. O. Truss, M.D., one of the authors, explained that fungus may play the leading role in symptoms and diseases such as allergies, gastrointestinal and bladder problems, fatigue, weight gain, and even "brain symptoms" like headaches, poor concentration, and irritability. Dr. Costantini's work also found evidence that mycotoxins caused rheumatoid arthritis.[2]

If you have not had success with your arthritis treatment, talk with your physician about this research and request that he or she prescribe any one of the several systemic antifungal medicines for a few weeks. While taking these, you must also avoid foods that would feed the fungi in the joints. Simply stop eating sugars (including those in dairy products, oranges, and melons), potatoes, and beans (including peanuts) for a month or two. If successful, you might want to terminate the drugs and try herbal antifungal remedies. Either way, your success will demonstrate to you and your doctor that the cause of *your* arthritis is no longer listed as "unknown."

References

1. Schumacher, H. Ralph, Jr., M.D. (Ed.). *Primer on the Rheumatic Diseases* (9th Ed.). The Arthritis Foundation. Atlanta, Georgia. 1988.

2. Costantini, A.V., M.D. *The Fungal Mycotoxin Etiology of Human Disease.* Johann Friedrich Oberlin Verlag. Freiburg, Germany, and Costantini, A. V., M.D., *The Fungal Mycotoxin Conference.* Toronto, Canada. 1994

3. Brown, Raymond Keith, M.D., et. al. Candidiasis: The Scourge of Arthritics. *The Townsend Letter for Doctors.* 911 Tyler Street, Port Townsend, Washington, 98368-6541. January 1995.

"Healthy Days are Here Again!"

A Testimonial
by Debbie O., Dallas, Texas

Our daughter was diagnosed with bacterial meningitis when she was 14 months old. It is common with this kind of meningitis for infection to settle in the joints. In Julie's case, it was her left elbow that was to be infected. After 14 days at the hospital on intravenous antibiotics, we finally came home ready to forget the previous three weeks. Fortunately, Julie returned to our family as a happy, healthy little girl, with the exception of a total hearing loss in one ear. Each year we saw an orthopedic doctor to be certain that the infection and her slightly enlarged elbow did not abnormally affect the growth of her arm.

All was well for ten years. After turning 11, Julie began to complain that her elbow was sore. We assumed that this pain was related to a change in the weather, or a bump, or a fall. Several days passed with no improvement, and we decided to make an appointment with an orthopedic doctor. After observation, X-rays, and Advil for a few weeks, it was decided that she should have an MRI.

The results of the MRI determined that Julie suffered from synovitis, which is a condition where fluid collects in the sac surrounding the elbow joint. The recovery and rehabilitation were very slow, painful, and frustrating for an 11-year-old and her parents. Unfortunately, the doctors were never able to determine what caused the inflammation in the elbow.

Just when we thought rehabilitating the elbow would mark an end to our ordeal, Julie began experiencing joint stiffness in different areas of her body. Most of the pain was in her neck, right index finger, and right ankle; however, some days her knee or her hip would also bother her. The stiffness, besides limiting her physical activity, affected her emotionally. Needless to say, we were worried and frightened by this unexplainable condition.

After another trip to the doctor, countless questions, blood tests, and a visit to a pediatric rheumatologist, she was diagnosed with juvenile rheumatoid arthritis. We followed conventional medical advice and through many tears, conversations, and lots of reading, decided to put Julie on a non-steroidial anti-inflammatory drug. Unfortuantely, it did not help. It was then suggested that we "needed to be more aggressive with our approach." The next step was a more potent anti-inflammatory and gold injections. Everything we read made us more disheartened and disappointed. What we were reading and hearing made us think that we would be doing more harm than good.

It was at that point that we made a desperation call to Doug Kaufmann. A friend of ours had mentioned Doug's work and encouraged us to call him. After talking with Doug on the phone for a few minutes, he gave us our first real hope since our personal nightmare began.

After visiting with Julie, Doug and Dr. David Holland told us that her problems might be yeast related. Dr. Holland prescribed an antifungal medicine and placed Julie on a restrictive diet. After two weeks, she felt 99% better. Once again, Julie was able to walk around easily and resume her normal physical activities, pain free. Most importantly to us, she donned her sweet smile. Julie continued on the diet for another month and, while it was not easy, it sure beat the alternatives! For the first time in seven months, Julie felt and acted like a happy, healthy 11-year-old — thanks to the wise counsel and commonsense advice of Doug and Dr. Dave.

Chapter Three

Fungi and Digestion

Intestinal disorders and fungi

Doug A. Kaufmann

As the title indicates, I am expounding on intestinal problems in this section. There are those of us who feel that seemingly harmless prescriptive drugs (i.e., antibiotics, cortisone, and birth control pills) can alter the terrain of the bowel enough to initiate an intestinal yeast infection. So often the intestines are the first tissues that are damaged by these activated yeasts, or fungi. For that reason, I thought you should learn how to identify whether your gut problems are really a serious disease for which you are relegated to a life of medicines, or whether your doctor may have been unaware that intestinal fungus can mimic serious intestinal disorders.

What serious gut diseases can these gut yeast infections mimic? Of equal importance is that you understand that the portal of entry of these disease initiators is, in this case, the mouth. Not only is there significant evidence that molds and their myco-toxins occur in our food supply, but once these devious little mold spores become activated (remember, antibiotics can activate them), everyday foods within our diet may feed them and keep them proliferating throughout the intestines. Of course, once flourishing within our intestines they can make life miserable. In these cases, it is quite common to have bloating, belching, intestinal gas, constipation, diarrhea, indigestion, and esophageal reflux. You can imagine what happens when these fungi escape the intestines via a "leaky gut" – a condition that is actually common once these fungi become active in the intestines.

Crohn's disease and irritable bowel syndrome (IBS) are very serious intestinal disorders. The dictionary states that sections of the alimentary (digestive) tract become inflamed, thickened, and ulcerated with these diseases. Crohn's disease is also known as *regional enteritis*, *regional enterocolitis*, and *inflammatory granulomatous bowel disease*. I will never understand why one set of symptoms had to be called by four different names, but such is allopathic medicine! You do not suppose that a disease so complex as to have four names might actually be a fungus in the gut and not really a disease at all, do you?

Two testimonial letters in this chapter are very thought provoking. I would not say that either case is cured of bowel disease; however, both found significant relief in addressing an underlying fungal condition. I often wonder what would have happened if I had met these people *before* the gastroenterologists met them. Could I have prevented further deterioration of the bowel? Was surgery really necessary? What role did carbohydrates or antibiotics play in the beginnings of their gut problems? More than their wonderful letters, I have begun to love both of these contributors and I thank them for the courage in apprising others of the fungal link to their diseases. Could fungus be contributing to your stomach and intestinal problems also? You bet it could!

The saddest part of these debilitating gut diseases remains that many gastroenterologists have absolutely no idea that there exists a fungal pathology in many cases of Crohn's and ulcerative colitis. By treating a pathogen (fungus) rather than a disease, it is very likely that many patients with gut diseases will get better faster. And most importantly, if a fungal condition exists after a short course of antifungal medicines, the patient can initiate an antifungal herbal approach. You might want the doctor to prescribe a systemic and gut antifungal medicine for a few weeks just to ascertain whether your gut problems are really a serious gut disease or fungus. If you feel better within two to four weeks, get to a health food store and inquire about natural antifungal remedies.

"Mycotoxins"
— fungal byproducts found in food

Patrick Kwan, M.Sc.

I have been following Doug Kaufmann's theory of the possible link between fungi and certain health disorders with interest for several years because I believe that what he says makes a lot of sense. When Doug asked me to write an article for him, I was slightly taken aback and jokingly asked him, "What does a food scientist know about fungi?"

Doug replied, "You must have a lot of dealings with molds and yeasts in your work with food products. Just think about it. I'm certain that you know more about fungi than you think."

After pondering Doug's suggestion for a while, I decided that Doug was right. I do deal with mold and fungus in my business … or should I say it deals with me!

I almost got into medical mycology (the study of fungus) when I first started graduate school years ago. I was already a licensed medical technologist specializing in microbiology, and it always intrigued me that nobody seemed to be concerned with or knew much about fungi and their relationship to human beings, except for vaginal yeast infections. Partly because I could not find a good mentor in medical mycology, I ended up studying food science.

Back in the early 1970s, **aflatoxin** was one of the growing concerns for food scientists. It had first come into prominence in the early 1960s when several flocks of turkeys suffered from acute *aflatoxin* poisoning in England. Yes, large doses of this fungal poison can cause death, even in people! In this case, over 100,000 turkeys died of aflatoxin poisoning. Later, scientists would learn that the aflatoxins that caused the deaths were traced to peanut meal in the turkeys feed mix. It turned out that the peanut meal was stored in an old silo with a window on one side. As the sun beat down on the feed mix through the windows, evaporation occurred and the resulting moisture migrated to the cooler side of the silo, away from the sun. The increased moisture on the cool side then allowed the mold *Aspergillus flavus* to proliferate and produce the mold poison called aflatoxin. Since that time, much research has been done on aflatoxin and its tumor-causing effects on human beings and various fish and animals.

The actual risk of these fungal poisons in our food supply might be higher than we think. Literally any whole grain or nut, if not handled properly during production and storage, may lead to mold growth and, therefore, mycotoxin production. Besides aflatoxins, food scientists are also concerned with **ochratoxin**, which causes kidney function disorders. It is produced by *Aspergillus* mold found commonly in soil and commodities like grains, nuts, beans, coffee, fruits, and tobacco; **patulin**, which is mutagenic and carcinogenic as well as acutely toxic, comes from *Penicillium* mold found commonly in soil and many fruits including apples (apple cider has been implicated several times) and even dairy products and meats; **zearalenone**, which has been implicated in estrogenic disorders, is a byproduct of a *Fusarium* mold which is very common in grains, corns, and even tomato plants.

There is no doubt that aflatoxin receives and deserves the most attention from the government agencies and the food industry. This is because of its common occurrence (especially in ground nuts) and its carcinogenicity. Once this mold poison is in a product, it is very difficult to remove without destroying the product. Even very high temperatures, as in roasting, would only reduce its level slightly. Basically, the maximum level of aflatoxin allowed by the USDA is 15 ppb (parts per billion), which is about as far down as scientists can go in detecting its presence.

I will never forget when I began working in the food industry. I was paid to crawl inside hot, stuffy boxcars to sample peanuts for aflatoxin. And I do mean SAMPLE! Sometimes I had to take up to 48 one-pound samples per lot. You see, out of a bag of peanuts, there may only be a few contaminated nuts, and I really had to make sure that a statistically valid number and size of samples were taken. Then I would mix and grind 48 pounds and take a sample for testing. Can scientists guarantee 100% aflatoxin-free nut products by testing? Not really. Unless I used 100% of the peanuts for testing, I would never guarantee a 100% non-toxic product. Obviously, this is not practical!

As the good doctors are now saying, prevention is the key to everything. To minimize aflatoxin contamination, we relied on very tight controls during all stages of the production of grains and nuts. This included proper agricultural practices to ensure dry conditions in the field and minimize mechanical damage to the kernel as well as proper storage conditions after harvest. Climate obviously played a big role during this whole process. Most importantly, communication at all levels was essential so that each player along the line knew what to observe in the product. Laboratory testing was only the last line of defense.

Are food products in the market safe from mycotoxins? I would say a qualified "yes." The safety record thus far has been very good. Will anyone guarantee it? Absolutely not. That said, peanut butter and roasted nut products on the market from reputable suppliers are quite safe from aflatoxin because every batch is usually tested either at the raw ingredient or finished product stage — and often at both stages. If you buy nut products, especially peanut butter, from a small supplier, make sure that the supplier knows what he or she is doing. Shriveled and discolored nut kernels as well as cracked kernels should be avoided.

Grain testing is not done as vigilantly as nut product testing. Although the risk for mycotoxin in grains is smaller than in nut products and the safety record has been good, we should never let down our guards. When dealing with grains, use the same precaution as for nut products. You can never be too careful when it's your own health that you are dealing with. Like Doug says, "Your health matters!"

Inflammatory bowel disease and fungi

David A. Holland, M.D.

Crohn's disease and ulcerative colitis, although distinguished by well-known characteristics, are collectively known as **inflammatory bowel diseases** (IBD) in the medical arena. IBD is characterized by a host of symptoms such as diarrhea, abdominal cramps, rectal bleeding, weight loss, fever, and a host of extra-intestinal symptoms, including disorders of the eyes, liver, gallbladder, muscles and joints, kidneys, and skin. (*Journal of Musculoskeletal Medicine*. Nov. 1996. Pp 28-34.) Treatment is usually focused on relief of symptoms with anti-inflammatory drugs or surgery.

The cause of IBD remains unknown. With all of our advances in medicine, why do the causes of so many diseases remain unknown?

Some have implicated a viral etiology to IBD. In the medical journal *The Lancet* (1996. 348:315-317), Dr. Wakefield and colleagues found that three of four offspring in mothers that had measles during pregnancy developed severe Crohn's later in life. Of note is that recurrent antibiotic-resistant pneumonia preceded the Crohn's in every case. This is important because antibiotics are known to increase the risk of fungal infection.

Other scientists have found carbohydrates to be a possible culprit. Two of three worldwide studies found the average intake of carbohydrates (including bread, potatoes, and refined sugars) to be much greater in those who developed IBD than in those who did not (Heaton, K. W. *Inflammatory Bowel Diseases*. Allan, R.N., Keighley, M.R.B., Alexander-Williams, J., and Hawkins, C.F. [Eds.]. Churchill Livingstone, New York. 1990.).

In her book, *Breaking the Vicious Cycle*, Elaine Gottschall describes the cycle of intestinal mucosal injury, impaired digestion, malabsorption, bacterial overgrowth, and increase in bacterial by-products and mucous production which lead back to intestinal mucosal injury. We all know that antibiotics can alter the normal intestinal flora or bacteria. These bacteria usually keep in check the relatively small amount of existing yeast in the intestines. However, when antibiotics are taken for various purposes (and you can bet those kids in Dr. Wakefield's study were given plenty of antibiotics!), the normal protective bacteria are eliminated, and yeast growth goes unchecked. The resulting effects range from "mild diarrhea to severe *colitis*, or *systemic fungal* or bacterial dissemination" (Saadia, Roger and Lipman, Jeffrey. "Antibiotics and the gut". *European Journal of Surgery*. 1996. Suppl. 576:39-41). In Chapter 2, you read about the link between arthritis and fungus. When fungi become systemic from gut inflammation and the overuse of antibiotics, you can see how the whole body becomes involved in what doctors refer to as "gut diseases."

Still other scientists have directly implicated yeast with regard to Crohn's disease. Former World Health Organization expert Dr. A.V. Costantini has found that people with Crohn's often have aflatoxin, a fungal toxin (refer to Patrick Kwan's article), in their blood. Barclay, G. R., et. al. (*Scandinavian Journal of Gastroenterology*. 1992. 27:196-200) found that disease activity in patients with Crohn's was lower while they followed a yeast-free diet, specifically avoiding baker's and brewer's yeasts.

Over and over we have had patients with symptoms of IBD who have experienced incredible improvement once they followed a yeast free, low carbohydrate diet. We have been a little more aggressive, though, and have added antifungal medicines such as nystatin which seem to speed up the improvement by inhibiting any further fungal growth.

Chapter 13 of *Principles and Practice of Clinical Mycology* (Kibbler, C. C., et. al [Ed.]. 1996. John Wiley & Sons, Ltd., West Sussex, England.) deals entirely with fungal infections in the gut. They describe how *Blastomyces dermatitidis*, a fungus, can produce granulomatous lesions in the intestines. Interestingly, this type of lesion has also been seen in patients with

57

Crohn's disease. Another fungus called *Histoplasma* produced intestinal disease with symptoms such as diarrhea, weight loss, fever, and abdominal pain – sound familiar? The common lesions seen in the gut with this infection were "masses or ulcers mimicking inflammatory bowel disease or carcinoma." The authors concluded that *histoplasmosis* should be a serious consideration in an immunocompromised patient with signs and symptoms of IBD. Now back to the big word "immunocompromised," which means a weak immune system. We strongly disagree that you must have cancer or AIDS or be on chemotherapy to have a weakened immune system. Just smell the air on your way to work or look at our standard American diet (SAD). Could these be impeding our immune systems? Anyone who has been diagnosed with ulcerative colitis or Crohn's disease knows the misery these diseases can cause. Given the alternatives for treatment, we think it would be worth a trial on a good antifungal program that includes diet, antifungals, and perhaps even desensitization to the fungi.

Intestinal fungi and the diseases they mimic

Is it Crohn's, or is it fungus?

Doug A. Kaufmann

So you've just been diagnosed with one of the many intestinal disorders! Well, before you take another anti-inflammatory pill or consider surgery, you absolutely must know that there is a chance that the medical community may be misdiagnosing many gut diseases.

In 1983, the *New England Journal of Medicine* published a correspondence letter from four doctors at the University of Tennessee Center for the Health Sciences. These doctors had learned that psoriasis (a skin condition that dermatologists do not know the cause of) and Crohn's disease (an intestinal disease that gastroenterologists do not know the cause of) may both be caused by yeast. Imagine that! One of the doctors, E. William Rosenberg, M.D., had previously discovered serendipitously that while treating skin diseases with the antifungal drug nystatin, several of the patients also had their Crohn's disease symptoms reverse. The doctors said, "We suspect, therefore, that gut yeast may have a role in some instances of psoriasis." And the same with Crohn's disease! How right they are, but why have 14 years gone by without making this important announcement?

Long before 1983, I learned that the Tennessee doctor's statement above was absolutely true and I set out to reverse these terrible diseases. Although I have been successful in doing this, I have been unsuccessful in teaching doctors about this incredible discovery. But why should I even have to try? Why aren't gastroenterologists receiving the life saving information that many gut diseases are really just fungal diseases in disguise? Could the answer be associated with the money trail?

Recently, I was invited to lecture to a group of Crohn's and colitis sufferers at a local hospital. Just before I was introduced, the man in charge handed me a brochure dispensed by all chapters of the Crohn's & Colitis Foundation of America (CCFA). It was entitled, "Questions and Answers about Diet & Nutrition." To make a long story short, this brochure stated very clearly that there was no special diet for these diseases and no foods worsened the symptoms. And who do you suppose would have produced this brochure? The very industry that has a vested financial interest in keeping people with intestinal diseases on medicines! This brochure was produced by a grant from a pharmaceutical company that produces drugs to treat the same, intestinal diseases!

A personal story of healing

A testimonial
by F. G., Fort Worth, Texas

I moved to Texas in November 1982, and all was well with my health until about two years later (1984) when I started developing allergies. These allergies got to the point where I started getting sinus infections almost monthly. Every month I would go back to the doctor and get another round of antibiotics for these infections.

After about a year of this, I went to see a specialist and he discovered polyps in my sinuses. Although he surgically removed them, my sinus infections persisted. Once again, I found myself going to the doctor for more antibiotics. I finally went to an allergist and started getting desensitizing shots and prescriptions for decongestants, antihistamines, and topical nasal steroids. This did not help with my chronic sinus infections, so he offered me, you guessed it, antibiotics!

During one of my infections, I didn't feel like eating much of anything for three days. No one had told me that when you take the combination of antihistamines, decongestants, and antibiotics, you should always eat — I learned the hard way. After sitting at my desk for five hours, I began to get light-headed and my heart started racing. This put me in the emergency room and I spent three days in a cardiac care unit. Luckily, I didn't have a heart attack, but I went through all of the testing, treadmill, stress thallium, echo cardiogram, and finally the cardiac catheter. Although my heart checked out fine, I continued to feel terrible.

For several years after that, I continued on the same routine with regard to my health: chronic sinus infections and antibiotics. This process would continue until 1993 when I discovered blood in my stools. After numerous trips to my primary care physician, I was finally sent to a specialist. They determined I had "antibiotic colitis." They prescribed cheese and yogurt. For six months my symptoms cleared and then they began again. Again, I returned to my primary care doctor numerous times and again he referred me to another specialist. I waited three weeks for an appointment. During this time, I really thought I was dying! Now chills, fever, and diarrhea were everyday occurrences. The specialist did a colonoscopy and diagnosed me with ulcerative colitis. He prescribed Prednisone and sulfasalazine to help control the symptoms. This initiated a long roller coaster ride. My health suffered and my symptoms returned with a vengeance.

In November of 1995 I was hospitalized for a week because of dehydration, loss of blood, and severe abdominal pain. I had heard of a person who owned a health food store and later learned that they could recommend some natural products that might help me with my condition. The same day the hospital released me, I went to the health food store. There I was loaded up with more than one hundred and fifty dollars worth of natural products. After reading all of the directions, I was supposed to take approximately 40 pills per day at various times and drink three different kinds of herbal concoctions. I attempted to stay on this program, but it caused my symptoms to worsen.

The following month I was back in the hospital for another week. The doctor notified me that if my condition did not improve within a few days, he would recommend surgical removal of my colon. The next day, the surgeon who was slated to do the surgery came into my room and detailed the surgical procedure for me. Fortunately for me, the 200 plus milligrams of Prednisone I was receiving in my IV started to work and I was able to put off the surgery.

At this time, I felt that surgical removal of my colon was inevitable, so I thought it was important for me to talk with others who had had this surgery. I was able to attend a support group meeting for persons with ulcerative colitis and Crohn's disease.

This meeting would turn my life around.

The guest speakers at this meeting were Doug Kaufmann and Dr. David Holland. They talked about the effects of antibiotics on the digestive system and of fungus within the colon. I soon realized that there were many similarities with my condition.

The following week I made an appointment to see them. Dr. Holland went over the restrictive diet program with me and prescribed some antifungal medicines that I needed to take. The following day my wife and I began the diet. To be honest, the first three days were almost unbearable, but after that I got used to eating the foods. During the first two weeks I noticed that the abdominal pain that I had lived with for the past three years was completely gone! My stools were completely normal and I felt better than I did before I was diagnosed with ulcerative colitis. An added benefit to this diet was that I have taken off four inches from my waist, my blood pressure has gone down considerably, and my sinuses are clear. I can't pretend to completely understand this process, but I cannot argue with the results. I can thank Doug and Dr. Holland for giving me a normal life again!

Treating
an "incurable" disease

A testimonial by Russ J.

I was first diagnosed with Crohn's disease at the age of 14, a little over 20 years ago. Since then, my primary symptoms have been diarrhea and anal fistulas. I have been on and off a variety of medications: Prednisone, Azulfidine, Asacol, Rowasa, Flagyl, and Cipro. I have had a total of six surgeries, which altogether removed about two-thirds of my colon or large intestine. Many of these things helped for a period of months or even years, but then my symptoms began to reappear or even worsen. Sometimes my fistulas got so painful that I began carrying a "fanny cushion" (made for hemorrhoid sufferers) with me everywhere I went and I took daily sitz baths.

At the beginning of 1996, I first heard about the Specific Carbohydrate Diet (SC). On the internet, I read testimonials of people who had been cured using the diet. My wife and I read a book that explained a low carbohydrate diet in detail and it gave many good recipes. I subscribed to a free, electronic mail Specific Carbohydrate Diet discussion/support group. This proved to be a great source of encouragement, information, and additional recipes.

In March 1996, my wife and I started the SC Diet. I began to see good results within a few days. After about ten days on the diet, I found myself having four to six bowel movements per day rather than the 10 to 12 I had previously had. Over the next few months I saw continued progress. I could often make it through a nine hour workday without having to "go." Prior to this diet, I went three to five times during the workday. Eventually my fistulas cleared up enough that I was able to get off both Flagyl and Cipro, which had been specifically pre-scribed to treat them. My wife's seasonal allergy symptoms seemed to get much better. This diet was really working great!

However, after ten months on the diet, I still had one persistent anal fistula and was still not having "normal" bowel movements. I had seemed to reach a plateau. I was much better than before the diet, but was frustrated that I saw little, if any, additional progress. I started listening to Doug Kaufmann on the radio, and he discussed the role of *Candida* (a type of yeast) in many diseases, including Crohn's disease. Doug and David Holland, M.D., were going to discuss this correlation at a local meeting of a CCFA (Crohn's and Colitis Foundation of America) sup-port group. I went and was impressed with what I heard. I made an appointment with them for the following week.

For two weeks they put me on a slightly stricter diet, which they refer to as an initial phase diet. Dr. Holland prescribed nystatin, an antifungal drug, and they told me to begin taking daily doses of psyllium hulls. This is a source of non-digestible fiber available at health food stores. Several of the 100+ members of the SC Diet e-mail had suggested the same things. As I had been warned, my diarrhea got slightly worse for the first few days on the program as yeast in my system began to "die off." By day ten on their program, I had the first normal bowel movement I'd had in several years!

Since then I have been able to reduce by 1/3 the dosage of Asacol (an anti-inflammatory drug) that I have been on for 18 months. A week ago, Dr. Holland prescribed Diflucan, a systemic anti-fungal drug, which we hope will help my one persistent fistula. Apparently, nystatin does not get into the blood stream, so it might be unable to reach the fistula. Again, I experienced some yeast die-off upon starting Diflucan, but that reaction seems to have subsided now. I am looking forward to seeing continued progress.

Many people in the medical community see Crohn's disease as an incurable disease that remains undaunted by diet. My experience seems to prove otherwise. I thank God for leading me to the help that I needed.

67

Chapter Four

Fungi and Respiration

Respiratory disorders and fungi

Doug A. Kaufmann

In our lives there can be nothing more fearful than the inability to breathe. Having one's airway constricted so tightly that suffocation ensues is frightening. Many believe that Jesus suffocated on the cross. This was the price He paid for our sins. Why must millions of Americans suffer so terrible a fate every day? And why do Americans suffer more than any other people in the world with this affliction? The answer will amaze you!

I read with awe and disbelief the May 1997 issue of *Life* magazine. The cover was entirely dedicated to respiratory distress. But it sells a ray of hope to readers. "If you are one of the 50 million Americans with allergies or asthma," it reads, "now you can take control of your life." The hope offered is based upon "new discoveries, smarter drugs, and breakthrough therapies." All of which, of course, we've been hearing for the past 50 years. Hmmm, now wait a minute. Fifty years ago, antibiotics were first introduced to America's children. It just couldn't be that simple, could it? Because doctors and researchers would have already figured that one out! Read on.

The central article in the Life Magazine issue of which I speak focuses on a four-year-old boy with asthma who loves the color, blue. "He drinks blue soda pop," it reads, "picks the blue marshmallows out of his Magic Star cereal, and grabs the blue crayon." Do you think even *one* physician who examined him saw a link between his asthma and the dangerous, blue dyes or the sugar in the food he eats? My guess would be "no!"

In their defense, medical doctors have licenses that preclude them from acknowledging anything medical except what they learned in medical school. This, despite their own Hippocratic oath which recites, "I will use dietetic measures whenever possible." Should a physician question, for example, that the antibiotics previously used on this boy might initiate or exacerbate his asthma, he would stand a chance of being reprimanded by the medical board in his state. Drug companies pay a great deal of money to medical schools and medical researchers. A fiduciary relationship exists between the senior medical staff and the providers of income streams. So, for a physician to even question that those providing money might in any way be involved in keeping Americans sick and in hospitals is un-American and unthinkable! And don't you even *think* of implicating chemical dyes in respiratory diseases. Remember that drugs are chemicals and chemical companies make blue dyes.

If I were a "fungally informed" physician, the first thing I would do is to tell the parents of the boy in the Life Magazine article to immediately change his favorite color to *orange*. Get him off the blue food he is eating, and get him drinking organic carrot juice every day. Carrots alone might improve his breathing condition, because I'm certain it's been caused by a fungus called *Candida albicans*. You see, a 1988 *Journal of Microbiology* paper maintains that carrots contain an ingredient that damages the cell walls of *Candida* organisms.

Now, how did *Candida albicans* manage to impregnate the lungs of the boy of whom I speak? More than likely, a prolonged round of antibiotics combined with his favorite foods — all high in sugar — caused the fungus to run amok in his intestines, from which it invaded his blood stream, enroute to the lungs. *Bronchopulmonary candidiasis* was the eventual result.

At any rate, I would encourage the boy's parents to obtain a prescription from their doctor for nystatin suspension, 100,000 units/ml. Nystatin is a harmless antifungal derived from a soil fungus. I would have the boy's parents administer this medicine following the morning and evening meals. I would educate them that if a fungus has gained access to the boy's lungs, it is living, it is parasitic and it requires food from his diet. I would inform them that foods such as soda pop and cereals feed the fungus and allow it to spread. At some later time in his life, it could possibly infect other tissues than just his lungs . Doctors who understand these dangerous fungi have reported their presence in *every tissue in the human body*. Many are only found at autopsy, when it is too late.

What upset me more than the content of this *Life* magazine article was the fact that I smelled a skunk! The article appeared to me to be nothing more than a sales pitch to get more unfortunate pediatric recruits for the National Jewish Medical and Research Center in Denver. Don't get me wrong, I'm certain there are wonderful medical people involved with this prestigious center. But I also know that each needs a paycheck. And just how do they get this paycheck? The insurance company of the family of the boy in the article paid $17,000 for a ten day visit! The boy went in with asthma, he went home ten days later with asthma, and it only cost $17,000! Medical mediocrity at its best!

Do you think it would have worked for this hospital to have a physician sit down for two hours with the parents in question to counsel them to change their son's diet, and to inquire as to whether the asthma got its start after a round of antibiotics? The question is, *worked for whom*? It would likely have worked for the sick boy's family, but it wouldn't have worked for the hospital, at least in terms of the profits it raked in from the insurance company. I will never understand why powerful insurance giants allow their money to be flushed into the medical institutions the way they do.

I am relatively certain that those in power in these insurance companies really do believe that they are doing the right thing. And if they want to throw away their money, far be it from me to challenge them. But when all their money is gone, watch them crawl into health food stores for relief for the stress they've self-imposed.

Patients remain sick, insurance companies continue to waste money, and hospitals and their staffs keep the profits flowing. Is it any wonder that we in America continue to suffer?

Is it asthma, or is it fungus?

David A. Holland, M. D.

Harrison's Principles of Internal Medicine, 12ᵗʰ Edition, defines asthma this way: "A disease of the airways that is characterized by increased responsiveness of the tracheobronchial tree to a multiplicity of stimuli ... manifested physiologically by a widespread narrowing of the air passages, which may be relieved spontaneously or as a result of therapy, and clinically by paroxysms of dypsnea, cough, and wheezing. It is an episodic disease, acute exacerbations being interspersed with symptom-free periods."

Is it possible to make something so complicated that we miss the simplicity of it? As with other diseases we have previously covered in other publications, the cause of asthma is often unknown. With a few cases we are able to pinpoint the cause, whether it is a chemical that is inhaled, causing lung damage, or an environmental dust like cement that can irritate the bronchial linings in the lungs and trigger wheezing and bronchial spasms in the worker, or victim. Once again, we will be looking at the role of fungus in this disease. We may as well include allergies, also known as allergic rhinitis, along with asthma in this discussion.

Often patients have both asthma and allergies, and the allergies can sometimes trigger the asthma or simply cause the daily misery of sniffles and congestion that you know if you are unfortunate enough to have experienced allergies. We hope to offer some simplicity to a disease that is approached with so much complexity.

I recently reviewed an overview of asthma prepared by a pharmaceutical company that was entitled, *Asthma Market Overview*. So, asthma is a market. A source of millions of dollars in profits. I guess that's okay; after all, we all have the opportunity to make a profit in this country. It is the people with asthma who fail to take an interest in their health who will continue to contribute to this market. Obviously, you are not one of these people. You have decided to stop the money trail by taking an interest and learning more about your particular condition. Whether this information helps you or not, we deeply appreciate the effort you are making to recapture your health. Let's look at some of the figures mentioned in this asthma report:

"An estimated 15 million Americans suffer from asthma, including 4.8 million children and adolescents."
(CDC. *Asthma mortality and hospitalization among children and young adults — U.S. 1980-1993.* MMWR)

"The prevalence of asthma is increasing substantially (38% over the past decade)."
(CDC. *Asthma – U.S. 1980-1990.* MMWR. 1992:41:733-735).

I wonder if 38 percent more antibiotics have been used over the last ten years.

"The total estimated cost of asthma in 1990 was $6.2 billion, up 38% from 1985."
(Weiss, K. B., Gergen, P. J., Hodgson, T. A. "An economic evaluation of asthma in the United States." *New England Journal of Medicine.* 1992. 326:862-866).

Based on these figures, whoever helps people substantially with their asthma is going to make a lot of money by taking the market share and upsetting the pharmaceutical companies at the same time! Overall though, they will be contributing to significant savings in both therapy and lives. Often we forget that there is human life behind all of these figures.

And then there was the *Life* magazine issue that Doug mentioned in his article "Respiratory Disorders and Fungus." There are two references in this article that I would like to expound on. First of all, it is widely known that sugar has the ability to depress the immune system. Anyone with a potentially fatal illness (around 5,200 people still die of asthma each year) should not be gambling with blue soda pop and Magic Star cereal. Cane sugar is a notoriously moldy food, and when consumed is able to introduce molds and their toxins directly into the human body. Speaking of mold, the article also refers to another asthmatic child whose former home tested positive for mold. Some mold growing in homes has been known to cause respiratory diseases and even bleeding from the lungs. Based on this observation my question might be: should the boy have been moved out of the moldy house more quickly, or should he simply have been prescribed more medicines to reduce the potentially toxic effect of the mold on his respiratory system?

An article by Kauffman, H. F., et. al. ("Review of fungus-induced asthmatic reactions." *American Journal of Respiratory Critical Care Medicine.* June 1995.) outlines the ability of fungus to not only cause an allergic reaction by simple exposure to the lungs, but also *colonize* the lungs and induce an inflammatory reaction from the infection. How common is this? A different Dr. Kauffman states that, "each year in the U. S. the fungi *Histoplasma capsulatum, Blastomyces dermatitidis,* and *Coccidioides immitis* cause more pulmonary infections than bacteria." (Kauffman, Carol A., M.D. "Nonresolving pneumonia: Is endemic mycoses to blame?" *The Journal of Respiratory Diseases.* Vol. 16. No 11. Nov 1995.) According to C. C. Kibbler, these fungi "routinely infect persons with apparently normal immunity" (*Principles and Practices of Clinical Mycology.* 1996. John Wiley & Sons, Ltd.) Ever notice that the asthma you once had as a child is no longer bothering you as an adult? It is well known that sensitization to fungi is higher in the early years and declines rapidly as we age (Kauffman, H. F., et. al.). If fungal infections, then, can contribute to asthma and allergies, why not treat asthma, when the cause is unknown, empirically as if a fungus caused it?

In a study on allergic broncho-pulmonary aspergillosis, a fungus-induced condition that can essentially mimic asthma and is a common complication of cystic fibrosis, **100%** (six out of six) of the patients treated with the antifungal drug Sporanox experienced improvement in lung function (Dennis, David W., et. al. Adjunctive Therapy of Allergic Bronchopulmonary Aspergillosis with Itraconazole. Chest 100; 3:813-819. Sept 1991.). This was a small study done in 1991. No interest in a larger study has occurred so far.

Another so-called "cause" of asthma, you may have been told, is reflux (that is, reflux of acid from the stomach up the esophagus and back down into the lungs, causing irritation of the lining of the bronchioles). Can this really be fungus as well? You guessed it – the most common cause of *Candida albicans* bronchopneumonia is from aspiration of oral secretions. Everybody aspirates a small amount of either oral secretions or stomach fluids at night while sleeping. If large amounts of yeast can cause pneumonia in a debilitated person, can it "just" cause asthma in a normal person? The question would be, is the acid causing the lung irritation, or is it the yeast that is sneaking in along with the fluids? And if it is the acid, what is causing it to reflux in the first place? We should not even have to answer that question!

We once saw a prominent man who had asthma and was spending upwards of $600 a month on asthma medications. He lived in a small town in Texas and, because of his frequent trips to the pharmacy, he had become good friends with the pharmacist.

In desperation and in light of not seeing any improvement after much time, he sought our help. We advised a particular diet known to starve fungi (vital to the program), a few supplements, and empirically, like the above study did, prescribed antifungal medications. The results were no less than dramatic. He lost weight, looked younger because of that, and was able to shed all of his asthma medication. The only dissatisfied party was the pharmacist, who no longer returned his phone calls.

Bronchial politics: how and why "asthmaphobia" was created

Doug A. Kaufmann

Why did two of the most established magazines in the United States, *Life* and *Newsweek,* devote their entire cover page to asthma in May of 1997? Could this be a public relations move on the part of the American Lung Association (ALA)? And just who are these folks that dedicate their lives to the well being of American lungs? Charities are often the public relations entities for the medical communities that they represent. According to the book *Unhealthy Charities,* you'd be surprised at who these "charities" are charitable to. About 13 years ago, one of my employees lost her father to cancer. My worst nightmare came true. I received a letter from her requesting that in lieu of flowers I make a "charitable contribution" to the American Cancer Society (ACS). Call it what you may, to this day I feel that my donation made a Porsche payment for a "cancer expert" affiliated with the ACS. Why is the grieving and bereavement process made socially acceptable in America only if a donation is made to a charity?

I, for one, will never ever donate another dime to a medical charity. Less than five percent (5%) of the funds raised by the ALA for "urgent need" research actually goes to any research at all! The other 95% apparently covers costs, including payroll. According to the above referenced book, the ALA is a marketing wing for the respiratory organizations, purportedly including doctors, who treat lung problems. So why all the PR on asthma? They're just doing their job. The more frightened parents they recruit into one of these hospitals, the more awareness is generated. Then it's just a matter of educating the parents on the wonderful job that the hospitals did to save their children's lives. Seemingly, a donation to the very charity that saved their child's life and then educated them on the complexity of breathing would be fitting. It's all marketing, kids!

So why should charitable money be invested in trying to figure out what causes respiratory diseases? Because medical institutions only make money when we're in them! It is my opinion that in their effort to keep us ignorant, they are making a few sloppy mistakes. The *Newsweek* article on asthma, for example, stated that "with the rise in vaccines and antibiotics, people in developed countries have experienced fewer serious childhood infections than ever before." Yet a survey published in *The Journal of the American Medical Association* reported that children receiving the pertussis vaccine were six times more likely to develop asthma than those not receiving the vaccination. And one only needs to review medical mycology to know that antibiotics can actually cause asthma. If it were true that our medical breakthroughs, i.e., antibiotics and vaccines, had reduced the number of asthma occurrences in America (certainly a "developed country"), how might you explain the fact that asthma rates have dramatically increased in every age group since 1982?

I believe that what irritates me most is the fact that the medical associations via their promotional and purportedly "non-profit" associations, seem to be preying on children. That is apparently their "target market." The mentality seems to be, "It's done with cigarettes, why not with asthma?" Each of the magazines mentioned above has small, helpless children on the cover.

Have you been watching the news or reading the newspapers lately? It seems that we have yet another medical epidemic on our hands. This one is called diabetes. It is now called the "hidden killer," because many of us have it and don't know it. And if we don't get to a doctor, we may die! Well, I predict that if this ad campaign for asthma doesn't increase hospital revenues enough, very soon asthma and other respiratory diseases will be billed as "toxic time bombs" ticking away in our children. And all of this is done in such a way as to make you feel that their concern is genuine. Indeed, I've long felt that most medical people have very high integrity, and remember: they are not to blame. But I am concerned about the integrity of those who have found that the secret to making money in medicine is through confusion and deception...scare tactics, if you will. Simply put, there are many to whom you are worth considerably more sick than when you are well. Your job is to use your head when consuming medical products or services.

I would never allow any one diagnosis to dictate my next move with my children. First, I'd see a medical doctor, followed by a health food store owner, followed by a chiropractor, followed by a nurse, and lastly a good (the good part is sometimes the most difficult) nutritional expert. I would never be fooled into believing that credentials in lieu of experience "made" the health care provider. Every day thousands of children are prescribed medicines for asthma by people with wonderful credentials; but I have known health food store owners who have amassed far safer and more logical treatment plans than chiefs of medical departments. Next, I'd take all of the knowledge that each person provided and I'd find someone I trust to help me with my decision. Knowing all of this should allow you, and your child, to breathe easier – and without a bill for $17,000.

A personal story
of healing

A testimonial by MFE, Plano, Texas

After I first met Doug Kaufmann, I finally began to see the light at the end of the tunnel. I cannot believe how much better I feel. Thanks to him, I have a life again. My only regret is not having met him earlier in my life and been given the ability to take charge of my life and my health.

Looking back over my medical history makes me realize just how long I suffered from *Candida albicans*. Over the years I was misdiagnosed by so many medical doctors and professionals that it is ridiculous. I realize now they treated the symptoms of my disease and not the problem, often masking the real problems with drugs. My whole way of thinking has changed so drastically that I will never trust my health in their hands again!

Back in 1972 I was diagnosed with asthma. I had always thought of asthma as a childhood disease, yet I was 16 years old. I was given expensive pulmonary function tests to measure and regulate the function of my lungs. I was treated with drugs, bronchial inhalers, and strong steroids.

From this point forward, I found myself shifting from one health crisis to another, never realizing until now that it was all connected to a fungus in my lungs. While my health continued to fail, the most dangerous focal point was always my asthma and lungs. Anytime I got the slightest cold or flu, I was prescribed a round of antibiotics to eliminate any further accumulation of fluids or germs in my lungs.

Around 1973 to '74, I began taking birth control pills to help regulate my menstrual periods and eliminate the painful abdominal cramping that accompanied them. I was also given strong pain medicine for the cramping. Today, I do not even need Tylenol. My asthma began requiring additional medical attention and stronger doses of the already prescribed medication.

In 1978, my medical doctor informed me that I would never live to be 40 years old because of my severe asthma.

In 1981, I married and on my honeymoon I got diarrhea that lasted four to five months. As I was euphoric, I passed this malady off to eating rich foods and making lifestyle adjustments. Again, medical doctors gave me enough drugs to stop the diarrhea to the point of constipation. No medical tests were run.

At this point in my life, I was a young professional woman at a high point in my career. I traveled, never exercised, and drank heavily – eating whenever I could. I paid little attention to any damage incurred and had my doctor's phone number memorized. He had even given me his private number for convenience reasons in case of emergency, as he considered me a regular patient with chronic asthma problems and the clock was ticking! He had already told me that I did not have long to live.

From this point, I was always the first one to have a cold, infectious bronchitis, and the flu. All I ever had to do was call my doctor who happily treated me over the phone, convincing me I needed a prescription of antibiotics to clear up any chest congestion, which would eliminate further complications. It would be true to say that I relied on my doctor heavily and trusted him to take care of my needs or this cycle would not have continued for as long as it did. I do not mean to blame everything on my doctor, but I was brought up to find a good doctor and then trust in him completely for all of my health needs. I even depended on him for referrals to other physicians when needed.

In 1983, I quit taking the birth control pills and became pregnant. During this period of time, I seemed to be relatively healthy. It was great! Other than some morning sickness during my first trimester, I enjoyed my pregnancy. Although I was big, I felt beautiful and very healthy. Following a normal vaginal delivery and nine months of nursing, I unfortunately resumed taking the birth control pills.

In 1986, I began to have chronic fungal problems under my toenails and was referred to a general surgeon for laser surgery. While this surgery was considered minor, the doctor stated that he had never seen anything like this before and he took many pictures in amazement. I required several additional surgeries (at least three) as the fungal warts kept returning with a vengeance. After each surgery, I was given antibiotics and pain medication.

Also during this time, I was in a severe car accident resulting in spinal fusion surgery along with more pain medications, muscle relaxers, and antibiotics for infection.

In 1992, thrush symptoms began in my mouth. The center of my tongue was white and had a film or coating on it while the sides were swollen, cracked, and had sensitive white patches. I also had diarrhea. My trusted physician diagnosed me as having eaten too much cinnamon candy and placed me on a bland diet for two weeks.

In 1993, my periods began to become a bother again, although I was on birth control and pain medication. I was given stronger pain mediation and a series of sympathetic handshakes. Finally, I was referred to numerous doctors for various treatments before being diagnosed with endometriosis. I did not want a hysterectomy, which was the "normal" procedure to correct this problem. Three of four doctors I consulted wanted my permission for a total hysterectomy surgical procedure based on my symptoms alone. The fourth doctor agreed to an exploratory procedure, based on my apparent apprehension, before performing a hysterectomy. The results of this exploratory procedure were overwhelming! I had the insides of a newborn baby – pretty and pink.

My pain continued and the doctor stated that I had pelvic congestion due to lack of satisfactory sex with my husband. He sent me home with a package of birth control pills. He suggested that these pills along with regular sex with my husband would take care of any pain or problems I was having.

In 1994, I developed another set of symptoms that were diagnosed as depression. The phrase "all in your head" took on a new meaning. As I saw doctor after doctor, patience wore thin at my house. Before I knew it, I'd been placed on anti-depression therapy. One doctor actually came right out and said, "it's all in your head." In other words, he had no clue as to what was wrong with me or what to do about it, so I must be crazy.

In 1995, I sustained a minor car accident injury resulting in an accumulation (later discovered) of mold and mildew in the trunk of my car. At this point, my health deteriorated to the "point of no return." Remembering that several years earlier my "trusted physician" had predicted that I would not live to be 40 years old, I truly believed that his prediction was finally coming true. I was dying.

Although only 39 years old, I found myself buying, planning, and paying for my own funeral. My husband took us on a fabulous trip for our fifteenth wedding anniversary. I was very sick for the entire trip. I could not keep food in my stomach for more than 15 minutes and found it embarrassing to eat. This was in May of 1996. To add to my frustration, during this time my husband lost his job and we had no medical insurance.

Upon arriving home, my severe asthma and diarrhea were horrible. The medical professionals advised me to drink Pepto Bismol daily and take prescriptive medicine to relieve the diarrhea. To their amazement, nothing worked – not even the strongest medication they prescribed. I use the term "medical professionals" because I went to several, none of whom could help me. They ran all kinds of tests, took blood and stool samples, and found absolutely nothing wrong with me. I found it more frustrating than they did, probably because they had my money for their services yet each looked at me with skepticism, whispers, and frowns.

After another run-around with the medical professionals, God blessed me and I found Doug and Dr. Dave. I was a total mess. My body could not hold food for more than fifteen minutes. I could not sleep, I cried all the time, was irrational and hard to get along with. I am certain that my husband would agree with this statement. When asked, "How do you feel?" I had mixed emotions. I felt sorry for anyone who loved or cared for me. I had been an emotional roller coaster basket case for many years and had never known why. I had been irrational, hot tempered, and sick without reason time after time.

Someone once said, "Smile, smile, things are not too bad." I had forgotten how to smile. When asked, "What do you do for fun?" I really had to think: fun – what is that? Fun was a privilege I had not enjoyed for so long I had forgotten what it was. I cannot believe that my husband still found me attractive. Most men would have left me a long time ago.

I had prayed to God to give wisdom to the doctors who tried to help me, and I found Doug. My girlfriend had tried to persuade me to call him for quite a while. However, I was skeptical of anyone but a medical doctor. Looking back, I now feel like such a fool. Immediately, Doug identified my problem and taught me that what I had been eating was actually causing my health problems. I just couldn't believe it!

Within two weeks, my diarrhea was completely gone and I began a long journey of healing. The road certainly has been filled with bumps full of skepticism and criticism – especially to those who claim to love me the most. I began to experience what Doug referred to as "Herxheimer's reaction," more commonly known as the "die-off" of fungus.

Once again, I felt as if I were dying. My hands were shaky, my vision was blurred, my ears were ringing, I experienced numbness in my hands and legs, and I was depressed, disoriented and confused. Besides the extreme fatigue, my headaches persisted, I lost some of my hair, and I cried almost all of the time. I dropped out of college for lack of concentration skills, and I felt worthless. My complexion went pasty white, and the people around me seemed to stare at me as though I were a freak. Several times, I was told that I should find another doctor or seek another opinion. Thank God I did not. I stuck it out, and now those problems are behind me. I really feel that Doug saved my life or at least gave me a life back. I am forever grateful for him and his staff.

Dr. Holland became a great source of support and I relied on his medical guidance coupled with their treatment plan for recovery. On several occasions, I have slipped off the diet and found myself in respiratory failure needing immediate attention. Help was only a phone call away. I cannot thank you all enough.

Chapter Five
Fungi and
Mental Health

The link between fungi and brain disorders

Doug A. Kaufmann

While working with Dr. Everett Hughes in USC Medical School, I collaborated on a research paper that dealt with attention deficit disorders and its link to diet. The paper concluded that, indeed, diet was a factor in many cases of ADD. This information and years of study piqued my interest in abnormal brain reactions caused by food and fungi.

Many years ago *Life* magazine presented a visual exploration of the intricate areas of the brain. This issue went where no other issue, or magazine for that matter, had ever gone: literally inside the human brain. Once inside this issue, readers discovered that although the visuals were excellent and intriguing, scientists still knew little about what this mass actually did.

This information void still exists today. Yes, we know more than we did in 1960, but considering that this organ governs our thoughts, our understandings, and our intellect, it is surprising that 20th century medicine knows so little about the brain's interactions with other parts of our body, let alone our nervous system.

The research possibilities are limitless when dealing with the brain and the nervous system. And there are very few "knowns." In lieu of understanding how the brain works, let's evaluate how the brain might react to extraneous factors ... say, fungal organisms. The scientific literature speaks about *meningeal* fungi. The meninges are the three coatings of the brain and the spinal cord. Since it is well documented that fungi can enter the blood stream, it is logical that these fungi can impregnate virtually any tissues in the body, including the meningeal tissues. In 1996, a medical textbook entitled <u>Principles</u> <u>and</u> <u>Practice</u> <u>of</u> <u>Clinical</u> <u>Mycology</u> devoted an entire chapter to fungal meningitis. The "-itis" on the end of that word indicates an inflammation of the meninges. And just what caused the meninges to swell? Absolutely right — fungus!

I am probably guilty of being a bit of a literalist sometimes when it comes to long words and medical concepts, but it has always seemed to me that if yeast can make bread swell, it can certainly make organs like the brain and its billions of connected cells swell, also. As it turns out, <u>Clinical Mycology</u> is one of many books that implicate fungi in brain swelling. Exactly what happens when the brain and spinal cord tissues swell is yet to be fully understood, but it can not be good! Doesn't cerebral swelling cause some headaches? Since certain areas of the brain control appetite while others control behavior, couldn't swelling impact those two as well?

Researchers have discovered six relatively common fungi that can invade the spinal cord. One, *Candida albicans*, can cause problems anywhere in the body. Another, *Cryptococcus*, primarily invades the meningeal tissues. Doctors say that people with impaired immune systems generally end up with the most health problems when this happens, but I have to question whether this is true.

Sometimes when people follow a specific program to eradicate fungi from their bodies, their brain symptoms clear up. These are some of the most exciting cases you have ever seen. It is my humble opinion that many people who are relegated to a life of phobias, tears, and antidepressants may really have an underlying fungal root to their cerebral symptoms. There is not a magic pill, diet, or exercise program that will create overnight success. Rather, an all-encompassing program must be initiated. And it can safely be done while continuing on antidepressants.

This area of fungal proliferation is important. It is important to explore the relationship between aberrant behavior and fungus within the brain. The important consideration is whether brain problems are psychological or physiological.

Diet, dimorphic fungi and depression

Doug A. Kaufmann

Roses are red, violets are blue,
I'm schizophrenic, and so am I!

~~~

A man walks into a psychiatrist's office with a large frog on his head. The psychiatrist says, "My, you seem to have a significant problem." The frog replies, "Yes, and until I can get this growth removed from my belly, it's likely to become more significant!"

~~~

There are no shortages of puns or jokes directed at mental illness. True depression, however, is no joking matter. Nor, say the statisticians, is it rare. According to the World Book Encyclopedia, approximately 14 million Americans suffer from depression. And, on a monthly basis back in 1990, doctors were writing or renewing in the neighborhood of 60,000 Prozac prescriptions (*Newsweek*. March 30, 1990). Just imagine today's count!

All of this data suggests that there are no shortages of depressed people or doctors willing to temporarily erase their symptoms. When dealing with depression, the question that continues to perplex medical scientists is: If we are merely erasing symptoms of depression with medication, what are they symptoms of?

I do not believe that depressed people suffer from a deficiency of selective seratonin reuptake inhibitors (SSRI). Yet, Prozac is but one of these medications meant to ease depression – a few hours per pill. There are actually numerous SSRIs and antidepressant medications, all aimed at controlling a symptom. There's that word again: symptom. What is depression a symptom of? Could it be fungus?!

The purpose of this book is to tackle not only physical symptoms of fungal infections but mental symptoms as well, and to educate people about how to recapture the health that most of them once had and that a few have never experienced.

The fungal link
to depression

David A. Holland, M. D.

There is not one of you reading this who has not either experienced depression, or at least known someone who has experienced it. After all, depression is a normal, human emotion. In fact, the absence of depression in certain situations, such as the loss of a loved one, can be abnormal.

There are, however, different degrees of depression. That which we will be discussing is the degree of depression that is defined as a clinical illness. You see, just like diseases such as diabetes, depression is defined by clinical criteria, criteria which, while not obvious to the majority of people, nonetheless have important implications regarding treatment.

Clinical depression often brings catastrophic consequences with it. It can alter decisions we make regarding our personal and business relationships, decisions that can have a dramatic impact on the future. It can damage our self esteem, our quality of life and even our health. It can destroy marriages and lead to job loss, hopelessness and even suicide. In short, as Doug writes, clinical depression is no laughing matter.

In this essay, I hope to outline how cases of clinical depression may often be linked to a fungal infection. Unfortunately, I may not find one psychiatrist who agrees with me. I can but present some studies that offer a differing viewpoint concerning this disease that strikes one in 20 Americans each year.

I should make it clear that, if you believe you may suffer from clinical depression, you should immediately seek the counsel of a qualified, psychiatric doctor. And, if you are correct that you suffer from depression, bipolar disorder or schizophrenia, you should not delay beginning treatment. I simply ask that you continue to educate yourself on the facts of your condition from this point on.

In 1984, W. G. Crook, M. D., published in the *Journal of the American Medical Association* (JAMA) an article called "Depression Associated with Candida Albicans." JAMA is among a handful of the most respected medical journals in the world, but the idea of depression associated with a fungal infection apparently did not catch on.

Among the causes of depression, you will fail to find "diet" or "fungi" listed as even remote possibilities. With the exception of life changes or stress factors, the cause of depression is often linked with genetics, i.e., "it runs in the family." It is difficult, then, to try to answer the question of how a fungus might cause depression. What would a living organism have to do with the way you feel?

You may have read that fungi excrete substances called myco-toxins. These are chemicals fungi produce that kill or limit the growth of other organisms, such as bacteria, that compete with fungi for nutrients. You may also have read that *antibiotics* are actually mycotoxins. In other words, using fungi, we now manu-facture antibiotics in massive quantities each day for the specific purpose of killing bacterial infections.

If mycotoxins are in principle harmful, is it not reasonable to assume that some do more damage than others? For example, penicillin is a popular mycotoxin that is regularly consumed by humans. In the proper dosage, it is only powerful enough to kill bacteria that have invaded our bodies. On the other hand, if you ever happen to have the misfortune of being exposed to enough of the mycotoxin, aflatoxin, you will almost certainly develop liver cancer, among other things. Incidentally, some scientists would argue that even penicillin is not actually all that harmless.

If you ingest a moderately powerful mycotoxin such as alcohol, you likely do so expecting an immediate effect. Alcohol can kill you, given enough quantity and time, but it quickly produces behavioral changes even in small doses. During digestion, alcohol is broken down into smaller molecules. One of the chemicals in this degradation pathway is acetaldehyde. If you aren't familiar with this chemical, simply recall yourself or someone you know who has had a hangover. Yes, it is acetaldehyde you have to blame for making you feel so bad. At least now you have something to blame! So, what are we getting at here?

In an article in the *Journal of Nutritional Medicine* (1990. 1:33-38), Hunnisett, A., et. al., discuss the "auto-brewery" syndrome. This is a condition whereby carbohydrates ferment in the presence of intestinal microorganisms to yield, you guessed it, alcohol! You don't need to visit a local micro-brewery: you are a walking, talking one yourself! In this study, 69% of the patients who consumed 50 grams of glucose (less than two ounces), about equal to the amount of sugar found in one soft drink, had measurable levels of ethanol (alcohol) in their blood stream only one hour after ingesting the 50 grams of sugar. And what fungus is responsible for the conversion of sugar into alcohol? Right again – brewer's yeast!

If 69 percent of you are fermenting in your intestines every day when you consume potatoes, grains, or beans (carbohydrates), and you are getting alcohol as a by-product in your blood stream, that alcohol has got to break down eventually into the hang-over chemical we discussed above. How would you feel if you had to walk around every day in a constant hangover? Do you feel as though you *are* walking around every day in a constant hangover? If so, you more than likely suffer from depression.

Do you see where the chronic fatigue syndrome comes into play, as well as depression? If you were an alcoholic, you can deduce that it would be best to avoid not only the alcohol but also the excess sugars and carbohydrates in your diet, lest you continue to feed your body the fuel it needs to produce the alcohol.

What if alcohol were not your problem, "auto-brewery" or not? What if toxins were to contaminate the food you eat? It's not unheard of. For example, horses sometimes suffer from a disease called duodenitis/proximal jejunitis syndrome (DPJ). DPJ causes the animals to develop depression and severe gastric reflux. Schumacher, et. al. (Vet. Hum. Toxicology, Feb. 1995. 37 [1]:39-45), have looked at how the fumonism B1 toxin, produced by the mold *Fusarium moniliforme*, may cause DPJ. When horses in their study were fed fungus-contaminated grain, they suffered both intestinal and liver damage. Do you, also, suffer from depression and heartburn? It just might be a fungus in your case, as well.

Other mycotoxins, such as T2, vomitoxin, and aflatoxin, all found in mold-contaminated feed, are well known to cause decreased appetite and weight loss in livestock. Weight loss and appetite changes are symptoms typically associated with depression. Could exposure to fungi or their mycotoxins be a factor in your symptoms, as well? Until we test for them in the blood stream, we will never know. Please let us know if you find a laboratory in the United States willing to run such tests!

There are means by which fungi can directly invade the meninges, or the lining of the brain and spinal cord. Meningitis is nearly always associated with behavioral changes. Most resources will tell you that such an infection, like candidal meningitis, is a devastating and rapidly fatal condition, but other fungi like *Histoplasma* produce a smoldering infection than can endure for years (C. C. Kibbler. 1996).

If you recall the chapter on bowel diseases, you will remember that many people with conditions like irritable bowel syndrome or Crohn's disease have neurologic manifestations as well. Most commonly, they suffer from depression! Could invasion from intestinal yeast into the blood stream or production of mycotoxins by these abundant yeast be the reason for depression? Don't let anyone tell you that yeast cannot invade the blood stream from the bowels. A. G. Prentice (Mycoses. 32 [Suppl. 2]. 42-46. 1989) says that "even without any other predisposing factor, overgrowth of *Candida* in the gut will lead to invasion of the blood stream."

Studies and evidence aside, most people who seek help from alternative medicine practitioners like Doug display a loss of energy to some degree, and many have been previously diagnosed with depression. As far as I'm aware, nearly 100 percent of Doug's clients have responded favorably to changes in their diets and the elimination of yeast and yeast-contaminated products. Certainly, if it quacks like a duck and walks like a duck, it must be a duck! When people suffering from depression improve following diet changes and elimination of yeast, it cannot be mere coincidence. In other words, the cause of depression is not genetics, but either a poor diet or a fungus.

Bygone days:
A treatment for depression
that worked

Doug A. Kaufmann

In the late 1970s, I opened one of the very first laboratories in the United States that dealt with the disease process as though it were nutritionally based. By the second year of operation, our gross income exceeded $1 million. During this time, I worked around the clock. I ran tests, made sales calls, did my own books, and cleaned the toilets. Rarely was I home. To say I was stressed would have been a gross understatement.

A friend suggested that I take a supplement called L-tryptophan to relieve my stress. I began taking this small pill twice daily and the change was noticeable and incredible. No, my job did not lighten up, but it seemed as though my body was fully relaxed and life was more enjoyable. My brain began to work in unison with my body! Knowing that such a feeling could be addictive, I used the L-tryptophan on an "as needed" basis only, and it never let me down. I recommended it to thousands of people.

L-tryptophan works by causing a natural elevation of the neurotransmitter seratonin in the pineal gland of the brain. When this neurochemical is elevated, peace and calm are promoted. Thousands of medical documents have confirmed that, indeed, this simple amino acid found in milk, egg whites, and turkey assists the body in producing calmness. Many doctors and nutritionists began putting their patients on L-tryptophan, and several of my psychiatrist friends used it to treat depression in their patients. Most commonly, L-tryptophan was used to induce peaceful sleep and dreams. It was simply a wonder supplement. And then something horrible happened.

A foreign supplier of this harmless amino acid supplement shipped a tainted batch to the U. S. Some individuals got very sick while taking the supplement. Others died of a condition called eosinophilia-myalgia syndrome (EMS). All of the people who suffered and died were taking L-tryptophan supplied from the tainted batch from a company in Japan. The Food and Drug Administration (FDA) immediately ordered all L-tryptophan supplements, no matter who manufactured them, off the market. There were several safe suppliers. This move seemed harsh since more people continue to die each year from over-the-counter aspirin than ever died from the tainted L-tryptophan.

In a startling move, the FDA allowed pharmacies to continue carrying L-tryptophan, but no longer could American citizens get this natural supplement over the counter. The bottle I used to pay $7 for now became available only following a doctor's office visit and a $40 prescription – a $100 investment. Finding a physician sympathetic to their patient's self-medicating needs became almost impossible. Worse, physicians were warned of the extreme dangers of having their patients use this amino acid that had maimed and killed.

At exactly the same time, the FDA was finalizing their approval of a new drug that artifically elevated the pineal gland neuro-chemical seratonin. It seems as though this seratonin runs through naturally occurring cycles throughout the day. It is produced in higher quantities when you are resting and sleeping and lower quantities when active. What this new FDA-approved drug, Prozac, did was readjust this natural cycle and inhibited the "reuptake" of scratonin whenever the pill was taken. What neither this drug, nor any other pharmaceutical drug on the market, has been able to do is to stimulate seratonin naturally and safely.

One might guess, therefore, that L-tryptophan, available from health food stores without prescription, was a hindrance to the makers of a group of pharmaceutical drugs called selective seratonin reuptake inhibitors (SSRI). Man could not replicate what God had provided naturally. There are now numerous SSRIs produced by several drug manufacturers. With the safe and natural L-tryptophan off the shelves of health food stores, a billion-dollar pharmaceutical bonanza was created. Prozac was FDA approved only four days after L-tryptophan was taken out of health food stores.

That was some 13 years ago. Today, many physicians likely don't even remember the scare that was created. It is likely that if you educate your doctor on the safety of this amino acid, he or she may write a prescription for you. Remember that L-tryptophan has a nutrient co-factor and should always be taken with 25 to 50 mg of vitamin B6.

Whereas your doctor may have forgotten the scare, your pharmacist may be another story. Pharmacists have wonderful memories, and most will not even carry this simple amino acid for fear of hurting you. Imagine that!!! Call around and find a compounding pharmacist in your area. They will provide you with L-tryptophan.

L-tryptophan was a wonderful breakthrough for depression sufferers. It seemed very unusual to me that the FDA would pull something off of the entire market because one foreign batch was tainted. It seemed even more unusual to me that 96 hours later a billion dollar pharmaceutical industry was created based on the success of this remarkable natural amino acid.

> **Note:** Since the original printing of this book, Prozac's patent has expired and L-tryptophan has, once again, become available without a prescription. A coincidence?

Food, fungi
and the forlorn patient

by Milt Gearing, Ph.D.

Almost any mental health professional will openly admit that the physiological causes of depression are not well understood. We do not know exactly what enables many antidepressant medications to work for specific patients, although we do know that they are effective in treating depression. Why does any given antidepressant work for some depressed patients and not for others? Why do some antidepressants work for a while on many depressed patients and then quit working? There are plausible theories offered as answers to many of these questions, but none of these theories has been proven.

During my years as a clinical psychologist, I have seen many patients who present with severe depression. Some of these patients have responded extremely well to antidepressant medication, while other patients have not. Since I have started working with Doug Kaufmann, both for my family's health and the health of my patients, I have referred to him some of my patients who suffer from depression.

All of these patients had tried antidepressant medications and gained little or no relief from them. All had worked in psychotherapy and made progress, yet each continued to be weighed down with serious symptoms of depression.

These patients were taken off all antidepressant medications and placed on the Initial Phase Diet (IPD), a low carbohydrate antifungal diet and program. All of these people have since shown amazing improvement in their depressive symptoms and a welcomed return to a normal lifestyle.

How is this possible? Some research in recent years has actually discovered a link between depression and diet. One of the best articles on this subject is called "Carbohydrates and Depression" (Wurtman, Richard J. and Wurtman, Judith J. *Scientific American*. January 1989. Pp. 68-75). One of the diet-related links to depression discussed by this article involves the tendency of sufferers from "carbohydrate-craving obesity" to consume excessive amounts of carbohydrates in order to improve their mood!

Just the opposite is true according to other authors. The landmark article by W. G. Crook, M.D., called "Depression Associated with Candida Albicans" (discussed by David A. Holland, M.D., in his article in this chapter) described a direct link between food consumed (carbohydrates) and depression symptoms in Candida (yeast) patients.

While there are many causes and many effective treatments for depression, those patients who do not respond to conventional treatments and who do show Candida symptoms should consider the benefits that the Candida diet and antifungal program could offer them for their depression. This approach has worked wonders!

Pain, depression and fungi

A testimonial
by H. H., Dallas, Texas

One would probably say that I am a happy, confident individual. I have not always been, however, the confident person that I am today. My life has been a roller coaster of ups and downs. As a teenager, I suffered from depression and eating disorders. At 13, dealing with both ailments, I tried to commit suicide. In the later years of my teens and into my 20s, my mood swings and low self esteem cost me many jobs. Never did I link the two with the foods that I ate. As a matter of fact, I realized the relation to depression and irritability only two days ago!

I began seeing Doug Kaufmann to relieve painful tendonitis symptoms. After two weeks of following Doug's Initial Phase Diet, the tendonitis greatly improved. With the help of holiday baking I "fell off the wagon" for about 16 hours. Once I had my first bite of sugar, I began my binge. I ate, and ate, and ate.

121

Several things happened. I craved more food, my arm started hurting again, and my sinus problems came back again. Most importantly, that old depressed and irritable feeling that I have struggled with for so long came back.

That night and the following day I was extremely moody. Any little thing filled me with anger. I felt impatient, anxious, mad at my lack of control, and mad at my husband because he didn't do things the way "I" wanted them done. He and I had a little "tiff" because of my anger and sarcasm.

Looking back over this "challenge" day of eating sugars has helped my husband and me see the true meaning of the statement, "You are what you eat." He and I went back on the Initial Phase Diet immediately, and within just a few hours I could feel a difference. I can now focus my thoughts and my mood swings are gone.

Chapter Six

Fungi and Dermatology

Skin disorders
and fungi

Doug A. Kaufmann

Dr. David R. Weakley was a Johns Hopkin's medical school graduate and professor of dermatology at Southwestern Medical School. In 1988, Dr. Weakley and I began working together at Medical City Dallas — a very large medical building, hospital, and medical theme park all rolled into one. Within a short time, Dr. Weakley had two other dermatologists working in his office. All was well as I set out to learn more about dermatology and they set out to add nutrition into their rather large dermatology practice. We would work closely together for five years.

Dr. Weakley was astonished with the many symptoms over and above general dermatology that we were able to reverse when using a dietary approach to skin conditions. I recall him being concerned that dermatologists were able to fix migraine headaches, bowel problems, and depression. Had he crossed a line in medicine? How could a skin doctor fix arthritis — a joint problem? I remember telling him that first and foremost he was a physician who took an oath to help people. Second, it was his medical establishment that had decided to compartmentalize the human body. He should be proud of his new abilities to get people better, no matter what they suffered from!

But along with this new pride came politicking. I remember insurance companies withholding payments to him because he tested his skin patients for food allergy. Their concern must have seemed logical to insurance companies. Why not rub some cortisone on it and charge $35? I would argue that 100 visits at $35 each for prescribing cortisone actually costs $3,500 – and the problem hasn't been fixed! Yet, we were able to transcend routine dermatology in reversing not only skin problems, but also numerous other problems for which these patients saw many doctors!

Soon, Dr. Weakley began fighting back. He wrote many letters demanding payments for services that he had rendered. He then apprised the insurance giants that dictated his practice (this is quite common today) that the monies that they had been dumping in gastroenterologists, gynecologists, internists, and rheumatologists offices could come to a screeching halt. He had been able to fix all of those problems by incorporating nutrition into his practice. You would think they would be thrilled! Yet the financial harassment not only persisted, but actually accelerated.

Prior to his death in 1995, Dr. Weakley and I learned a great deal about the role of food allergies in dermatological conditions. We used a blood test to detect food allergies. Although today this is commonly done, in 1988 we were pioneers. Some years earlier I had discovered the root cause of most food allergy, and Dr. Weakley was impressed with these findings. During our first few years together, we tested patients for food allergy in order to confirm that they did, indeed, exist in dermatology patients. If so, Dr. Weakley would often write a prescription for antifungal medicines to test my theory. And why antifungal prescriptions for food allergy? You will find this interesting!

One of my mentors in medical science was Dr. Everett Hughes, with whom I worked on a limited basis at USC Medical School. We had collaborated on several research papers that Dr. Hughes had published. I did the food allergy tests, and he interpreted this data, along with other data he gathered, in an effort to confirm that food caused symptoms! One day after a pleasant lunch, Dr. Hughes asked me how food allergy could be so accurately detected in the blood. Did food actually get into the blood? We guessed that undigested foods somehow leaked through the intestine and ended up circulating in the blood. Although this sounded terribly illogical, it was the best that we had in the 1970s.

Some years later, I read a research paper entitled, "Antigenically intact food macromolecules exiting the gut lumen." This paper confirmed my suspicions that small pieces of undigested foods, still intact, leaked through tiny holes in the intestinal wall and gained access to the blood stream. Once there, a type of white blood cell (B-cell lymphocyte) recognizes the food particle as foreign, forms an antibody protein against the food, thus rendering it harmless from causing damage inside the body. After the food particle combines with the B-cell antibody protein, these tiny "micro-food-chips" are referred to as either "antigen antibody complexes" or "immune complexes." These complexes are then filtered out of the body.

As the years have passed, I've stopped worrying about food allergy. Yes, it does exist and yes, I am one of the individuals credited with starting the "food allergy revolution" in the 1970s. But testing for food allergies is, in my opinion, not really necessary anymore. I am less concerned about food leaking through the intestines than I am with my concern as to why holes exist in the intestinal wall. And what about the normal inhabitants of the intestines leaking out? Remember that there are yeasts and bacteria inside the intestines and should these be allowed to cross the intestinal barrier, problems significantly worse than food allergy would soon surface.

Septicemia is the word used to describe blood poisoning by bacteria. *Fungemia* applies to fungus gaining access to the blood. In either case, doctors will sound the alarm when these conditions are known or even thought to exist. Now I am certainly not a doctor, but I have always wondered how bacterial infections spread, if not via the blood stream. And I have often pondered why antibiotic and antifungal medicines are **systemic medicines** (actions occur by the medicines crossing the gut-blood barrier and the blood-organ barrier) given the general medical consensus that these microorganisms would kill a person if they ever got into the blood. Yet I constantly hear, "My doctor said that fungus could never get into my blood stream because it would have killed me if it had." I dare say it is confusing!

You will find that *septicemia* and *fungemia* are most likely quite common, unbeknownst to most physicians. In 1963, Harold Hyman, M.D., the prominent author of a medical encyclopedia, stated that approximately one-half of the population of the United States had suffered from a systemic fungal disorder that had largely gone unnoticed.* How could this be if fungus would kill a person if it ever gained access to their blood stream? Has the population of the U.S. decreased by 50% since 1963, or have medical doctors learned wrong information in most medical schools? Hmmm.

Finally, while we're on the subject of skin, just how many skin conditions do food and fungi cause? I believe *all* of them, but you'll be hard pressed to find one dermatologist who credits *any* skin symptom or disease to food or fungus. Do skin patients really suffer from steroid medication deficiency after all? I would challenge any physician and certainly any specializing in dermatology, to take the Kaufmann challenge. Yes, I believe that acne, rosacea, psoriasis, dandruff, hives, and eczema, to name a few, intimately link food with fungus. No, the dermatological organizations do not concur.

* Hyman, Harold. The Complete Home Medical Encyclopedia. 1963.

The science
of skin fungus

David A. Holland, M.D.

As you already know if you've been listening to Doug, the skin is the largest organ in the body. It serves many functions, the least of which is to protect you from outside invaders. Most importantly, it keeps our insides from becoming outsides! Everything is neatly tucked into our body by nature of the skin. What you may also know, then, if you are a faithful Doug Kaufmann "roadie," is that the skin may serve as a signal of deeper processes occurring inside of your body. In fact, skin lesions are at times the earliest clue to the fact that one has a systemic mycoses, or internal fungal infection (C. C. Kibbler, 1996).

Part of the claim to fame of fungi is that they were actually the first microorganisms shown to cause an infection or disease in humans. Specifically, it was a fungus called *Trichophyton schoenleinii* (you'll be quizzed on this later!) that caused skin infections in humans (*Principles and Practice of Clinical Mycology*. Kibbler, C. C., John Wiley and Sons, Ltd. 1996.). This being the case, you'd think that everyone would know about the ubiquity of fungi. Not so, however. Southwestern Medical Center, one of the most prestigious medical centers (in our area, at least), touts the fact that they receive $150,000,000 annually in research grants, yet they do not staff *one* mycologist among their hundreds of scientists and physicians. It is a similar story across the country: not many mycologists actually exist. It is no wonder that the role of fungi is often overlooked and that the extent that fungi play in skin disease is commonly unknown.

One of the more familiar groups of fungi is the dermatophytes. These usually cause only superficial infections, such as "jock itch" or toenail fungus. A dermatophyte infection of the skin is also known as "ringworm." Fungal infections of the skin are one of the most common infectious diseases in the world with an estimated 10% to 15% of the entire world's population being infected with these (C. C. Kibbler)! The sources of these fungi are many: soil, animals, human contact, and plants.

Sometimes these supposedly superficial infections can cause symptoms in parts of the body distal to the part that is actually infected. For example, one may have a terrible athlete's foot or toenail infection and then suddenly break out in a rash on the palm of the hand. We call these "id reactions." The rash on the hand is not due to the athlete's foot, but rather from the myco-toxins (fungal poisons) released by the athlete's foot fungus into one's bloodstream. These, in turn, affect the palms of the hands. The palm rash is due to the toxins, not the foot fungus, per se.

There are other ways that skin fungi are able to affect the body internally. Through a non-official poll, we found that many patients with toenail fungus coincidentally also had elevated blood cholesterol levels. Then, once the toenail fungus was treated with an antifungal, the cholesterol reduced! (British Medical Journal. 1995. 311:919-22). By deduction, this would mean without a doubt that the fungus contributed to the high cholesterol. Costantini (1994) has found research explaining how fungal toxins (mycotoxins) exposed to the blood stream caused an elevation in that person's blood cholesterol as a protective measure: cholesterol binds fungal toxins, thereby rendering them less harmful. Get rid of the fungus, then, and your body won't need the excess cholesterol.

On the flip side, we have seen how internal fungal infections contribute externally to skin diseases and symptoms. Persons with coccidiomycoses or blastomycosis (infections of the lungs) may suffer from a variety of skin lesions. Some may even resemble skin cancer (C. C. Kibbler)! *Candida albicans*, a yeast that is found in nearly every single normal, healthy person, can not only cause external skin infections, like diaper rash and perleche (manifested as dry, red, cracked skin at the corners of the mouth), but it may also contribute to internal problems like vaginal yeast infections and intestinal problems.

There are still other skin diseases, like psoriasis, acne, hives, and eczema, which don't seem to have such an obvious relation to any internal infection. However, people have been treated empirically (treatment based on experience vs. evidence) for internal yeast or fungal infections and have the external problems go away as well. There is a collection of literature showing that psoriasis is indeed a fungal infection, caused by either the fungus itself or, as we discussed above, caused by the fungal toxins released into the blood stream (Costantini, 1994). This literature has been supported by many personal testimonials of people who were treated for fungal infections and were "cured" of their psoriasis. (I used the quotes because psoriasis is supposedly incurable, but I beg to differ!)

The internal problem in most cases is preventable. Usually it is caused by a diet high in refined carbohydrates and yeast foods and/or exposure to certain drugs, like antibiotics, steroids, or birth control pills. For example, I have yet to meet a child who suffers from eczema who hasn't also been exposed to antibiotics in one way or another at an early age. At other times, the internal problem has been a result of inhaling fungal spores and succumbing to a systemic fungal infection, regardless of how healthy you were to begin with. Remember, an external, fungal infection can always be a sign that something more serious and devastating is happening inside your body. To that end, even things like toenail fungus should not be taken lightly.

If you happen to be one who suffers from a chronic skin ailment, especially if no one has been able to offer relief or cure, the possibility exists that you would respond to a combination of a change in diet and either natural or pharmaceutical antifungal remedies. As always, "you are what you eat." So, your diet is going to play the most profound role in long term relief.

The Kaufmann challenge

Doug A. Kaufmann

Now that we've whetted your appetite and piqued your interest, let me make a broad generalization about the medical field. In my 25 years of studying nutrition, I have never seen any one specialty in medicine that loves big words like I have seen in dermatology. To be perfectly frank with you, I can't pronounce them all, but I'll just bet that a good dermatologist can! The problem remains that there is a vast difference in the ability to pronounce big words and to cure big problems. Would you rather your dermatologist pronounce them or reverse them?

In his excellent dissertation on skin fungus problems, Dr. Holland mentioned that empirical evidence (the body's response to a treatment) sometimes proves stronger than logic. Again, please understand that the information here should never replace an initial physical visit with a dermatologist when you have skin problems. If that doctor gives you the clean bill of health or recommends a treatment that you are not comfortable with, please tell him! Many of you will have positive results with this program, and that may well be the way to educate doctors!

Imagine if three or four of their patients called them back and said, "This is something you need to learn!"

Here's how I'd begin investigating the role of food and fungus in my skin condition, if I were an otherwise healthy adult:

1. Unless otherwise directed by a physician, eat only meat, poultry, fish, vegetables (no potatoes, corn, or beans), green apples, grapefruit, berries, eggs, nuts (except peanuts), and seeds. Eat no sugars, bread, grains, or pasta.

2. Drink eight to ten ounces of fresh-squeezed organic carrot juice twice daily and in this "cocktail" place one teaspoon of apple cider vinegar.

3. Take two caprylic acid tablets, three times a day.

4. Stop taking all unnecessary supplements and retain only those that are absolutely necessary.

If I had bowel symptoms, especially constipation, I'd take one heaping tablespoon of psyllium hulls in a small jar of water (4 to 5 oz.), shake well, and drink quickly. I'd do this each night just before bed.

This program may worsen the skin problem for the first few days, but continuation should cause remission within a short time. You might try this program for 30 days. Take a Polaroid picture of yourself prior to beginning, and then again in 30 days. If you see a vast difference (and are fully dressed!), share these pictures with your friends and doctors. You deserve to have great skin, and they deserve this information.

Chapter Seven

Fungi and Heart Health

The heart of the matter
... is it fungi?

Doug A. Kaufmann

Do you recall what you did yesterday? Fifteen hundred individuals cannot recall what happened in their lives yesterday — because they lost their lives to a heart attack. Thousands more are crippled each day from cardiac complications. Heart disease is the major cause of death in this advanced medical arena we call the United States.

There are no shortages of "experts" and published medical research papers confirming that cardiac disease is a killer. But if they are all right, why do the deaths and statistics just keep climbing? Are we not heeding their expert advice, or are the experts wrong?

Pick up any nutrition book, speak with any cardiologist, or call the American Heart Association — each will confirm that cigarette smoking, high cholesterol, and diet cause heart disease. You will not, however, find what I believe to be the true cause of heart disease from any of the "experts." Sometimes "experts," even in alternative health care, are blind when it comes to the cause of heart disease. A respected alternative medical book expounding solely upon heart disease was published in 1997 and features many prominent alternative physicians. Again, we see nothing more than a compilation of nutritional articles and nutritional therapies. There is not a word on fungus or yeast in this entire book. If you don't understand what causes something, your conclusions on how to reverse it are moot. Sometimes you stumble onto a treatment that actually works. You might now be wondering if natural cardiac strengtheners like CoQ_{10}, grape seed extract, and hawthorne berries are actually antifungals. I'm proud of you!

I believe that a sedentary lifestyle causes heart disease. Our bodies were meant to move! I agree that diet contributes to heart disease, but I disagree as to which foods in the diet are contributors. I believe that wheat, corn, potatoes, and sugar have far more to do with coronary disease than bacon and eggs. Although it is virtually impossible to find any one referring to this, I believe that alcoholic beverages cause more heart disease than pure, unadulterated dairy products (try to find those!). In essence, I believe that low fat diets being promoted by dieticians and heart associations are responsible for keeping them in business! Low fat means high sugar!

And cigarette smoking? In 1968, a researcher by the name of Bock discovered that fresh cut tobacco leaves did **not** induce cancer, but cured tobacco (a proprietary process used by the tobacco companies that purportedly adds yeast and sugars to the tobacco) **did** induce cancer. So it appears that the tobacco industry may be making their product hazardous to our health — even without their knowledge. And what industry could possibly win by having cigarettes so full of dangerous fermented yeast and sugar?!

Now you ask, "OK, Doug. What does cancer have to do with heart disease?" It is my opinion that the same thing that causes cancer also causes heart disease — and many other diseases in man. Since I figured this out many years ago, there has been nothing more frustrating than observing the actions of the American Heart Association (AHA), a fund raising organization that raises money by selling its name to food producers. Pick up a box of many of today's popular multi-colored or frosted cereals and you will notice a stamp of approval from the AHA. Do you sincerely believe that the AHA is acting in the public's best interest by "endorsing" these sugar laden products? It is time for Americans to stand up and realize that when money is involved there are smaller moral standards and larger bank deposits.

The powerful AHA is not alone. The American Cancer Society (ACS) and even the American Medical Association (AMA) have sold their names — in the public's "best interest," of course!*

145

We're on our own, kids. And we'd better learn how to take care of our heart health, because there is no shortage of for-profit hospitals that gleefully endorse these glorified fund raising activities.

If you suffer from any number of heart conditions, it is imperative to be evaluated by a physician first and foremost. Most likely, medicines and/or surgery will be prescribed. As it is in all areas of medicine, not just cardiology, it is unfortunate that many doctors have no concept of how invasive the fungal infections really are.

*The AMA recently rescinded its contract with Sunbeam, a manufacturer of medical products.

The heart of fungus

David Holland, M.D.

It seems these days that there are only two things to die of: a heart attack or terminal cancer. Granted, there are many more sad ways one can leave this cruel world, but on our healthy quest we probably think of these two ways as our prime enemies. I mean, these are what we want to prevent while on our mission to a healthy life, aren't they – along with a disease-free life and a quality existence? Preventing these diseases is something that is in my hands – my control, to the extent that God allows. And even then, who knows when I'll be struck down by a truck (I do live in Texas, remember). But while I'm here, I'd like to take my best shot at living a healthy life, wouldn't you?

Now, when we speak of heart problems, what do we think of most often? That big word "cholesterol," right? Haven't we been pounded into thinking that cholesterol has something to do with either preventing or succumbing to a heart attack? The trendy word for cholesterol is "fat." Low fat this and low fat that – I'm so sick of "low fat" that I'm beginning to experience chest pains. Years ago doctors recognized the fact that some people with heart problems, specifically atherosclerosis ("hardening of the arteries," from now on referred to as coronary artery disease, or CAD), had extremely elevated serum cholesterol levels. From then on, cholesterol became an immediate enemy. What is worse is that they assumed that if our serum cholesterol was high, we must have been getting extraordinary amounts in our diets – we were "pigging out!"

So, out the cholesterol came – excommunicated from good food as we know it. The question now is, "Does cholesterol, a natural substance found in every human cell, directly contribute to plaque in my arteries?" Did you know in over half of the subjects suffering from heart attacks, the victims had normal cholesterol levels? Enough of this: let me put down my fat free Hershey's Chocolate Syrup and let's tackle this subject.

I first direct you to the work of Professor A. V. Costantini, M.D., retired head, World Health Organization Collaborating Center for Mycotoxins in Foods, who took 18 years of his life, at his own expense, to dig up every article he could find on fungi, mycotoxins, and their relation to CAD. He put his collection together into a book (Fungalbionics: Atherosclerosis. 1994. ISBN #3-930939-00-2). Good luck trying to get this book here in the U.S. of A. It wouldn't be a very popular book with certain establishments here. In his conclusion of this collection, Dr. Costantini states, "There is a known cause of atherosclerosis and that cause is the fungi and their mycotoxins." He also summarizes that there is, indeed, a food relation to the cause of CAD, but it is only food that has been contaminated with fungi and/or the mycotoxins they produce. The information presented in this book is overwhelming, and way beyond the scope of our discussion now; but suffice it to say it puts the question of what causes atherosclerosis to rest.

One study in the *New England Journal of Medicine* (April 3, 1997) looked at the role of inflammation in the risk of developing atherosclerosis. As is typical, what was not addressed is what caused the inflammation! Always look for the cause, not for the sign or symptom. Also, when you look at or hear any new studies that try to address the cause, ask yourself, "Who funded this study?" Remember what I said above: Dr. Costantini researched for 18 years at his own expense, specifically without the funding of pharmaceutical companies. Week after week I hear well-meaning pharmaceutical company representatives present the latest studies on why their drug is better, only to disappointingly find out that their own company funded the study. What do you expect the results to be?! Certainly, they are not going to favor their competition.

What about taking a cholesterol-lowering drug to lower your cholesterol? If you are the less than one percent of people in the U. S. that genetically inherit a tendency to develop abnormally high cholesterol, I think it may be a good idea. Otherwise, I'd be asking you, what are you doing through exercise and diet?

How do these drugs work anyway? A study on one such drug, Lovastatin, showed that it inhibits fungal growth (Antibiot Khimioter. 1996. 41[11]:3-6). On a smaller level, the drug inhibits a certain enzyme involved in the manufacture of cholesterol; but did you know that many cholesterol-lowering drugs were initially studied for the purpose of killing fungi? Perhaps they were more profitable as cholesterol-lowering drugs. Fine with me, as long as they kill those fungi!

Should you even worry about severely high cholesterol? I would! Elevated cholesterol is a response to an invasion by a toxin in your blood stream. Remember Costantini's research (1994) explaining how fungal toxins in the blood stream caused elevated blood cholesterol: cholesterol binds fungal toxins, rendering them less harmful. Rid yourself of the fungus and your body doesn't need the excess cholesterol.

Does your doctor doubt this? Ask him or her what would happen if you took the drug cyclosporine, a drug used to suppress the immune system so your body does not reject an organ transplant. One hundred percent of the time you will develop elevated cholesterol and, subsequently, atherosclerosis -- and also, in some instances, cancer! Cyclosporine, folks, is a mycotoxin – a poison produced by a fungus and used as a drug.

Several mycotoxins are found in foods such as corn, peanuts, beer, barley, apples, and wheat. The steak you are not eating is less likely to be bad because of the meat and fat than it is because the cattle ate moldy feed, complete with fungal poisons. Those poisons are now stored in the fat! I'm not sure how to get around this to eat the meat safely, but fiber in vegetables do bind mycotoxins. So, be sure to eat fresh veggies or use a psyllium fiber supplement when you eat that meat.

"Don't they screen for toxins in grains?" you might ask. They sure do, and we know of one laboratory that does. But we do not have a zero tolerance for mycotoxins in grains in the U.S. It would be cost prohibitive. We only routinely screen for one of the several hundred known mycotoxins. You would nearly have to quit eating to completely avoid every source of mold and mycotoxin. But you can be wary of the more "notorious" foods like corn, peanuts, and beer. I will give you one hint on beer: they tend to use the poorer quality, often moldy, grains for producing beer. (Counsel for Agricultural Science and Technology. Report 116. Nov 1989.) Just think about that as you wonder why alcohol is implicated in so many diseases! And please, folks, unless you have one of those rare disorders with cholesterol, eat those raw nuts (all but peanuts) and eggs, like Doug keeps telling you.

A 1960 American Cancer Society study showed that those who consumed **more** than five eggs per week had *fewer* heart attacks and stroke deaths than those who ate **less** than five eggs per week ("Eggs are Great Food." Joseph Hattersley. *Townsend Letter for Doctors and Patients.* January, 1996). Another study in the mid-1970s concluded that you could cut your risk of heart attack by 50%—and 60% if you are a woman—by eating nuts five or more times per week. Naturally, we're not talking about the honey-roasted variety nor those roasted in peanut oil!

Let me give you my take on this: I am pretty convinced that oxidation in the blood stream or cholesterol in and of itself has little to do with atherosclerosis. The plaque which is responsible for causing blockage of the arteries and subsequent heart attacks is a complex formation of immune cells known as a "granuloma." Never mind the long word, but the formation of a granuloma in the body requires the presence of a foreign substance – either a "bug," like a fungus, or a metal or toxin, like a mycotoxin. Cholesterol is not a foreign substance. Neither is oxidation a foreign process, but rather one that is used by our body to perform normal, daily protective functions. And I do think that if you are a fervent exerciser it is okay to eat the right kinds of carbohydrates; but if you are either sick or are among the ranks of couch potatoes, I think that the ever-popular low fat, high carbohydrate diet is one of the most harmful things for your body.

Excess carbohydrates, which are, in simpler terms, sugars, are stored as fat inside your body. Declaring across the board that every one should eat low fat is to say that we are all equal. Look at the size and shape of different people. Do you really think one diet is right for every one of us? Of course you don't. That is exactly why there will always be a battle as to which diet is better. If you are unwell, though, I'd lose the carbs!

CASE PRESENTATIONS

The cases of three clients that Doug and I worked with several years ago appear on the following two pages. Please take special note of the numbers involved.

Case No. 1

We consulted with a 37-year-old male who had a triglyceride level of 342 (normal is less than 200) and a total cholesterol level of 237 (normal is less than 200). His HDL, or good cholesterol, was low at 30, while his LDL, or bad cholesterol, was high at 139. His doctor had advised a low-fat diet, weight loss, and more blood tests in two months.

After two months on the low-fat diet, tests showed that his triglycerides had shot up to 703. Although his total cholesterol actually dropped slightly to 224, his protective HDL had fallen even lower, down to 25. His LDL was not even measurable because his triglycerides were so high.

At this point we saw him, advised a high protein diet high in unsaturated fats (i.e., raw nuts and avocados) and low in carbohydrates. His trigliceride normalized within two weeks.

Case No. 2

We saw a man in his 30s with triglycerides over 1,000 and a cholesterol count of more than 300. Within ten days of starting our low-carbohydrate diet, his triglycerides had dropped to 160 (normal) while his cholesterol came in at 205.

Case No. 3

A 50+ year old male with cholesterol of 293 and triglycerides of 350 came to see us. Two weeks after starting the program

mentioned above, he had a cholesterol of 198 (normal) and triglycerides of 226 – well on his way to normal health.

Why I can't sleep late Saturday mornings

Nathan L. Lipton, M.D.

After working all week as a busy opthalmologist, I look forward to being able to sleep in on Saturday mornings. Well, Doug Kaufmann put an end to that! Several months ago, while lying in bed one Saturday morning, enjoying the freedom of not having to get up, I happened to begin listening to the radio. I tuned in to 94.9 "The Word," a station I often enjoy for its spiritual content. That's when I first heard the excited, enthusiastic voice of Doug Kaufmann blasting the medical profession for over-treating everyone with antibiotics and other assorted sins that we physicians commit. I quickly found myself listening intently and even agreeing with much of what I heard.

I am a board-certified opthalmologist in practice for 20 years. I treat patients of all ages and specialize in laser vision correction and surgery for cross-eyed children. But I certainly know that we doctors don't have all the answers. Because I am intently interested in alternative medicine, I have always been open to learning about all facets of health from whatever sources I could find. I had listened to other health and nutrition-oriented shows, but "Your Health Matters" was different! I knew I was hooked when, the following Saturday, I set my clock for 7:00 a.m. to catch Doug's program from the beginning to the end.

Although I feel that Western medicine as practiced in this country is the most advanced in the world, I have recognized for many years the importance of nutrition as the foundation for health. My two favorite quotes on this subject are:

The doctor of the future will give no medicine,
but will interest his patient in the care of the human frame,
in diet, and in the cause and prevention of disease.
— Thomas Edison

~~~~~

Our food should be our medicine.
Our medicine should be our food.
— Hippocrates

Besides being one of millions of Doug Kaufmann radio listeners, I have also gotten to know Doug as a friend. Not surprisingly, he is just as terrific off the air. What really comes across with Doug is his sincerity and how much he cares about helping people. For me, Doug also fulfills the role of teacher; I am constantly learning from him. I am honored to have been asked to contribute to this section.

Heart disease
and diet

Doug A. Kaufmann

Atherosclerosis means "clogging of the arteries." Like most diseases in America, the cause is unknown but the treatments are many. This chapter has been dedicated to every individual who has ever thought they were having a heart attack and really weren't. Had you known that the meal you just finished was actually the cause of those horrible symptoms, you could have relaxed a little. Instead, you went to the doctor, had a physical exam, and were informed that your heart was just fine.

Which diet is the best one to prevent the symptoms that mimic heart attack? Heart disease is often a symptom of a complex event taking place within your body. A parasitic fungus can gain access to your heart and circulatory system and cause irregular events within the body. Since the fungus is parasitic, it requires certain foods to feed it. Fungus craves carbohydrates like potatoes, pasta, and bread. So, the next time you pull your car off the road and worry about that impending heart attack, take a moment and review what you just ate. It is likely that this review will have you knowing that your diet must change!

Chapter Eight

Fungi and
Allergies

The fungal link
to allergies

Doug A. Kaufmann

The year was 1972. I had just been honorably discharged from the U. S. Navy after serving a turbulent, albeit rewarding, four years. I was now trained in acute care medicine. I was disillusioned because those four years had likely resulted in the loss of a formal medical education. I really did want to become a physician, but had neither the grade point average nor my youth to support me through medical school. I resumed my college studies in Los Angeles and began working with an ear, nose, and throat allergist. Dr. Howard Gottschalk was one of the finest men I have ever met in the course of my medical career.

Like health maintenance organizations today, the military herded patients through like cattle. At my tender age, I truly believed that this was as good as it got in health care. Dr. Gottschalk would provide the integrity catalyst that I so desperately needed to witness in medicine. He absolutely loved his patients and, of equal importance, they absolutely loved him.

I became certified by the American Society of Allergy Technicians (ASAT) in 1973 and worked with Dr. Gottschalk for six years in that capacity. He was a visionary who instinctively knew the future of medicine. Within two years of my employment, he sent me to the Washington University School of Medicine in St. Louis to research food allergy. Food allergy, mind you, was extremely controversial. Within a year of returning home from St. Louis, the allergists across the street from our small office would "educate" the public that food allergy was extremely rare, affecting perhaps only a miniscule percentage of the population. I am certain that we represented competition to them, and they wanted to squelch this concept of food allergy as quickly as possible.

You see, the concept of food allergy involves a resolution of two medical hurdles. If immune reactions to food *did* cause disease, the general public might be able to bypass a doctor's visit and recover by changing their diet. Simply changing dietary patterns would seemingly "cure" the affliction, if food allergy existed. This was unspeakable in 1975. No one could possibly self-diagnose! Additionally, doctors are not taught nutrition in medical school. If food really did cause symptoms and diseases, an admission would have to be made that something was sorely lacking in medical schools. I believe the term my sons use to dispel this notion would be "fat chance." As we all know, doctors learn *everything* in medical school!

The erroneous information that the allergists were dispensing never daunted Dr. Gottschalk, who was immune to perpetuating medicine solely for turf protection. For me, however, this was a new concept. Those of you who have followed my work through the years know that today I am undaunted by medical deception, just as Dr. Gottschalk was in 1975. Today, it seems, misleading the general public has become the standard. The miniature print on pharmaceutical drug advertisements, in my opinion, represents only one form of lying or deception.

Allergy is defined as an adverse reaction to an otherwise harmless agent. Food, animal dander, pollen, dust, and molds are otherwise harmless agents. Many allergists today still contend that food allergy is quite rare, yet most will skin test their patients for foods. I've often wondered why they do so, when their own academy denies that food allergy exists in all but a small portion of the population. Certainly, allergists cannot just be in it for the money! Most must really believe that food allergy is a problem, or they just wouldn't skin test for foods.

There is overwhelming clinical research to substantiate the *in-validity* of skin testing to diagnose food allergy, yet I do not know of one allergist who doesn't bill insurance companies for these inaccurate tests. Allergists have long fought blood tests for food allergies. This is because food immune responses are most likely due to the formation of different antibodies (a white blood cell's response to anything foreign in the blood stream – like a pollen) than airborne allergy and these cannot be detected on skin tests.

Skin testing can only determine one type of allergic response, which is rarely food induced. It is sad that the well being of the public is often disregarded when finances are at stake. It seems that much of the medical profession just doesn't appear to care about the truth. The mentality seems to be, "If a doctor orders a test, he must be right." Be careful out there!

This chapter will counsel you on trying to naturally relieve both inhalant allergies and food allergies. After all, do you really want to know what you're allergic to, or do you want relief? My friends, if we dare to overcome our allergies by ourselves, then we also dare to overcome our allergists by ourselves.

The cause behind many allergies

David A. Holland, M.D.

"I've never had allergies before I moved to Dallas!" the patient tells me. She speaks with a nasal voice and sniffles.

"How long have you lived here?" I ask.

"About a year and a half, now."

This is a typical scenario I encounter several times a week, and I'm just one guy, in one office. I wonder how many other doctors hear this on a weekly basis.

East Texas is the perfect place to develop mold allergies. There is humidity, rain, and the usual winds: perfect for disturbing the mold spores following the rains.

"My allergies get worse when it's raining or when it's humid," is another comment I hear frequently.

"Allergies" is a broad topic, and one that we had a difficult time narrowing down. You've got your classic sinus allergies or allergic rhinitis. This is also called "hay fever" and is accompanied by symptoms of sneezing, watery eyes, runny nose, etc. You've got allergies to drugs like penicillin (which, as you know by now, is a mold by-product). Then you've got asthma, skin allergies like hives and eczema – the list goes on and on. "Hay fever," by the way, was a term derived from the manifestation of fever after being exposed to *Aspergillus*-laden, moldy hay. You can already begin to see how fungus is inevitably tied into allergies!

Obviously we want to discuss further how fungus can be related to why you feel so miserable. Grab that box of Aloe Vera Puffs before you start. OK, now – read on!

Dr. C. Orion Truss, M.D., a pioneer in the work and study of candidiasis and its relation to various illness and symptom patterns, describes "the familiar manifestations of allergy" related to exposure to and infestation with the *Candida albicans* yeast. *Candida albicans* is one of the most allergic substances known and studied. See Dr. Truss's book *The Missing Diagnosis* published in 1985 and his article, "Tissue Injury Induced by Candida albicans," in the appendix of his book. Dr. Truss continues: "Once the mucous membranes become inflamed by their allergic response to yeast products, infection begins to occur with great regularity at random sites from the nose to the lungs."

Patients often come into the doctor's office not so much because of allergies but because of the subsequent infections that they cause due to the chronic congestion in the sinuses and lungs. At this point, antibiotics and possibly steroids are prescribed, both of which lead to further stimulation of fungal and yeast growth. Do you see how a vicious cycle can be created at this point?

R. J. Hay, in "Fungal Infections" (*Manson's Tropical Diseases*. Cook, G. C. W. B. Saunders, Inc. 1996. Chapter 59), informs us that hay fever or asthma due to molds like *Aspergillus*, *Alternaria*, and *Penicillium* species is estimated to account for *up to 15%* of respiratory allergies! That means one in six of you with hay fever may actually be infested with a mold that is causing your allergic symptoms. And you thought it was just because allergies run in your family!

An article in *Chest* (Adjunctive Therapy of Allergic Bronchopulmonary Aspergillosis with Itraconazole. Denning, David W., et. al. September, 1991. 100:3.) describes how **100%** of patients with severe asthma symptoms due to *Aspergillus* fungus experienced improvement in symptoms after being treated with an *antifungal* medicine called Sporanox, or Itraconazole.

Do you have chronic sinus infections, with or without aller-gies? CNN.com has reported that, in September of 1999, the Mayo Clinic maintained that "almost all cases" of sinusitis may, in fact, be caused by a fungus. The clinic reasons that this may be why "millions of sinus sufferers do not find relief from anti-biotics and nasal spray." What the clinic does not acknowledge is, if a fungus causes most cases of chronic sinusitis, then antibi-otics have only served to fuel this disease, in terms of financial loss and physical suffering. If this were the case, an antifungal program would be required to eradicate the disease. CNN re-ported that the clinic estimated 'it will be two years before any treatments are available." The year 2001 has come and gone — and the clinic has yet to propose a course of treatment.

How do you know if your symptoms of allergy or asthma are due to a fungus? You might consider trying an antifungal pro-gram with a changed diet and antifungal remedies and see if you don't feel much better. Your other option is to live an occasionally miserable, and sometimes life-threatening, exist-ence. Analyze what you might lose by trying the former. This is what Doug is talking about when he refers to "branching out" and educating yourself on your disease.

How about those of you with hay fever, allergies, or asthma in your childhood but you "grew out of it?" It is known that "sensitization to fungi is high in childhood and declines rapidly with age" (*American Journal of Respiratory Critical Care_Medicine*. June 1996. 6:151:2109-2115.). If you continue to have allergies as an adult, you can almost be certain that you are still having problems with fungi. I am convinced that childhood asthma has very little to do with genetics, dirty carpets, and cockroaches and more to do with diet, antibiotics, and molds.

I think that people with hay fever want to know if there is any hope and if there really is a "magic bullet" to rid them of their miseries. I can only speak of the number of people who walked into Doug's office with Kleenex in their hands, wiping their noses, and two weeks later were using the Kleenex for tears of joy because their life-long miseries were on the way *out* of their lives. Granted, none of those who did not put forth an effort shared in the joy. Changing the way you live and eat is no easy feat. But neither is living a life with allergies.

I am not an allergy specialist, and I have no interest in becoming one. I do expect some criticism in, perhaps, lack of scientific evidence as to how molds and allergies are linked. But, once you piece together the literature that *is* out there and know the right questions to ask your patients, it is evident that molds cause more allergies and asthma problems than a physician would ever imagine.

What *I'd* do
If *I* had allergies

Doug A. Kaufmann

I hope you carefully read Dr. Holland's section in this chapter, *The cause behind many allergies.* I believe that, unless you were to dig for many months, you would not find many articles at all in the scientific literature that implicate fungi as the cause behind allergy and asthma. But, neither would you find much work that links hyperactivity with sugar, even though many parents know this to be the case. You see, scientists are often very careful to hide truths that may injure their credibility or reduce their income. This may well be the case with some of our nation's allergy specialists.

Like all diseases in America, allergy is a progressive problem — it's getting worse every year. Allergy specialists, or *allergists*, struggle to understand this mysterious disease and the intricacies of an immune system that would allow seemingly harmless antigens, like cedar or elm pollen, cat hair/dander, or wheat, to wreak such havoc.

If I suffered from allergies, I'd probably find an *immunologist* at the local medical school who would help me to better understand my condition. Immunologists are not medical doctors; rather, they are immune system researchers. They receive doctor of philosophy degrees in immunity and are quite knowledgeable about allergies. I'd also try to find an ear, nose, and throat allergist as opposed to a regular allergist. ENT doctors, in my opinion, have a superior testing system (the Rinkle Serial Dilution System) and are more in tune to foods and fungus being the causes of allergies. I am of the opinion that foods and fungus are far more important to understand than are dust and pollen. You can often control food and fungus yourself! Turning your allergies over to a nurse giving two to three shots weekly means losing control over your condition. And you thought insurance companies really had *your* best interest at heart!

Based on my knowledge of allergy and immunology, if I suffered from allergies, here's what I would do:

First, I would get to a doctor and have a *Total IgE* blood test. Although a family doctor may run this test for you, I've found that allergists may not want to run this test. You see, the results of this simple, inexpensive blood test may cost an allergist hundreds of dollars in skin tests. Protective protein immunoglobulins (also known as antibodies) come in five classes. One of them, *immunoglobulin E*, known as the allergy antibody, normally runs from 0 – 150 in healthy, non-allergic adults. The problem for any allergist is that many of his patients who *appear* allergic have very normal levels of this immunoglobulin. Instead of trying to figure out this discrepancy, allergists often exclude the use of this blood test.

Please allow me to interject my limited knowledge regarding this blood test. It is my assertion that *most* people who appear to be allergic actually have either post-therapeutic dysbiosis (intestinal overgrowth of fungus or bad bacteria provoking allergies following antibiotics or other medicines) or mold allergy that will not elevate the level of IgE in their blood. In either case, allergy tests need not be done – in my humble opinion. Rather, I'd follow the recommendation listed below if my Total IgE was within the normal range.

Next, I'd change my diet to prevent fungal and mold growth. Most environmental fungi are saprophytic, meaning they consume dead and decaying material. Once inside the human body, however, they become parasitic — they require a host (that's us, kids) to supply them with food. They love yeast (baker's and brewer's) and sugar. They are not particular as to what form the sugar comes in, so fruits (fructose), table sugar (sucrose), all grains, breads, pastas, beans, and potatoes should be avoided due to their carbohydrate content.

If I had nasal sinus allergies, I'd use a nasal spray made from grapefruit extract such as NutriBiotic's "Grapefruit Nasal Spray." Grapefruit seed extract is quite a good fungicide and often fungi inhabit the nasal pharyngeal passage. This nasal spray costs only about $10 and I'd take two puffs three times daily for a few weeks to see if that helped.

A product made by Solaray called QBC seems to work well for allergic individuals. The "Q" stands for quercitin. This citrus bioflavinoid seems to block the receptor sites on allergy cells, thereby limiting binding of pollens. The "B" stands for bromelain, often used for inflammatory problems, and the "C" stands for vitamin C.

Herbs, used by people for centuries, seem to be specific to each individual case of allergy. Whereas one person can take *Eyebright* for eye allergies and have great results, another may have no results whatsoever. This can be logically explained by the toxicity threshold of each individual. A very toxic individual may have to detoxify prior to worrying about their allergies.

It is my opinion that one day science will find that literally any seed that survives the germination process is an antifungal. Fungus is so prevalent in soil that it engulfs and consumes many plant seeds. Those that it doesn't consume could become vigilant fungicides. Today, scientists have studied onion, garlic, and grapefruit, to name a few, and have found that these have fungicidal effects. Just imagine the magnitude of my hypothesis! Any organic food or herb could be used to control allergy, but only if the etiology of the allergy is fungus! Since many pharmaceutical drugs are derived from herbs, one could argue that pharmaceutical medicines work by eliminating fungal proliferation! And guess what? Many do! The point is, you will find numerous herbal remedies for allergic conditions and some sufferers swear by them. Just remember that the reason they work may have more to do with the etiology of a person's allergy (fungus?!) than the herbal remedy, itself.

The ecology of the intestines is crucial, and when this is out of sync (a condition called dysbiosis), allergic reactions can occur. If, for example, you've had horrible allergies since taking birth control pills, steroids, or antibiotics, it is likely that these pills could have altered the terrain of the bowel enough to bring about the allergies. This being the case, I'd try a wonderful product made by Natren. It is called *Healthy Trinity* and is a replacement therapy for the upper and lower intestines. Be careful, because not all good bacterial replacements are the same. Natren has stood the test of time and has very high quality ingredients.

When it is difficult to establish a basis for your misery, try increasing the productivity of your immune system. This is assisted with a nutrient called *Beta-Glucans*. The Seagate Company in San Diego has an excellent beta-glucans, which they mix with either organic carrot powder or pure shark cartilage. The NSC Company in Reno, Nevada also has an excellent beta-glucans called either NSC100 or NSC24.

I know that my frustration with the medical community can be discerned in my writings, but there really are doctors like David Holland out there. Many actually take an interest in their patients' struggles and are happy to learn that something other than traditional allergy tests and shots work for their patients. Most doctors, other than allergists, know that traditional allergy work-ups and desensitizing injections aren't the answer. Otherwise, they would send all of their allergic patients to allergists – something not many doctors do any more.

Most importantly, if you have a good relationship with your doctor, then know the importance of educating him or her as to what controls the allergic symptoms their prescription couldn't control! You'd be surprised how many doctors would welcome a nice letter from a patient informing them that *stinging nettles* relieved their allergies. And, who knows, perhaps his next cure could be thanks to you!

Please see our website for contact information concerning some of the products mentioned throughout this book.

Chapter Nine

Fungi and
Women's Health

Women's yeast-related health problems

Doug A. Kaufmann

What comes to mind when those two words, "yeast infection," are said? Vaginal yeast, right? This chapter will explore issues deeper than doctors are capable of! By the time you put this book down, you will likely have more knowledge than most physicians as to the significance of those two seemingly harmless words, "yeast infection."

Perhaps not all female health problems are generated by yeast or fungus, but once a determination has been made that a fungus is the cause of a woman's health disorder, inevitably the question as to how the microorganism entered her body should be explored. This can actually occur in many ways.

Once the fungal spores gain access, they can disseminate throughout the body quite easily via the bloodstream. Inhalation of fungal spores creates one portal of entry and often mimics asthma or any number of respiratory diseases. Sexual transmission of fungal spores is known to exist, as will be discussed later in this chapter. I believe, as do many other health professionals, that most fungal infections directly involve the use of broad-spectrum antibiotics. In my opinion, one of the first questions any medical practitioner should ask his patients is whether *any* symptoms began shortly after taking *any* antibiotic, thereby helping to confirm a cause and effect relationship. Although many women link vaginal yeast to antibiotics, more complex symptoms could and should be attributed to these medicines. Antibiotics as a cause of yeast infections have been very well documented for decades. Less understood, but of equal importance, is the causal role of hormones in yeast infections. Prescriptive hormones include steroids, such as cortisone, prednisone, and the birth control pill.

One interesting note, here, is a confirmation of my long-term hypothesis that yeast and fungi are directly linked to cancer. John Glaspy, M.D., medical director of the UCLA Joint Medical-Surgical Oncology Center, recently stated, "Theoretically, *all* hormone treatments/hormone replacement therapy (HRT), birth control pills, and fertility drugs can cause cancer." Since there is good evidence that all steroidal hormones can increase fungal overgrowth, this statement may finally add fuel to the fire of the link between cancer and fungi.

I feel compelled to apprise every woman of the fact that we have known for years that fungi can be transmitted sexually (Oriel, J. D., et. al. Genital yeast infections. British Medical

Journal. 4:761. 1972). Unfortunately, not much is published about this important phenomenon. Although I have no scientific documentation to confirm this, it appears that male alcohol intake plays a vital role in some female health problems. If I might venture a guess, I'd say that men who drink beer (grain, sugar, and yeast!) maintain a skin fungal condition that can be transmitted during sexual intercourse. These fungi remain dormant on the male exterior dermis, where the temperature is 70 to 80 degrees. Once a 99 degree mucous membrane tissue is involved, they seem to activate and proliferate. In the early stages, a woman might not notice any symptoms. Within a few days or weeks, these fungi may mobilize within the female reproductive tract, causing widespread damage including endometriosis, vaginal yeast, painful intercourse, and bladder infections. Remember when we called bladder infections "honeymoon cystitis?" Why did we know then but not now that female bladder infections were linked to a male partner? Not surprisingly, symptomatic relief often accompanies the use of appropriate prophylactic measures. You can now understand why I believe that men's prostate problems are directly linked to fungi. Fungal prostatitis has been reported in numerous scientific journals. Once fungus has been transplanted to the proper (female) host and becomes activated, the male is vulnerable to infection – not on the skin, as was the case when he was the carrier, but now within the urethra and the male reproductive tract. The urethra of the male passes directly through the prostate, which is exposed during sexual intercourse. In my humble opinion, anything capable of making bread swell just by adding heat and moisture is also capable of making *any* tissue, including the prostate gland, swell just by adding heat and moisture! Testicular pain is also a common complaint, as this yeast is exchanged between sexual partners.

What symptoms can fungi and yeast cause once activated within the female? I believe that the list is endless. Certainly, when one understands the danger of toxins produced by fungi, it is plausible to claim that infertility, miscarriage, painful intercourse, menstrual problems, false positive pap smears, lumps, cysts, and endometriosis, to name a few, could each involve fungi. Think about this fact: prepubescent girls have ovaries and a uterus, yet never have ovarian or uterine cysts or endometriosis! Why is that? A male sexual partner just has to figure in somewhere! Conversely, all boys have a prostate gland, but only men get prostatitis! Why does this fact seem so obvious to you and me, yet allopathic medicine has never even broached the subject?

For the record, I do not believe in mammography. This "business" of finding cancer early presupposes that we even know what cancer is. According to John Lee, M.D., since 1992, most pathologists have known that *"carcinoma" in-situ* duct cells *do not* progress to cancerous breast tumors; yet surgery, chemotherapy, and radiation done following this diagnosis create an illusion that mammography really works. I do believe, however, that mammography represents a very accurate breast fungal test. Even calcium oxalate deposits have been identified in tissues infected by some fungi. These truths may be withheld from the general public because of the sizeable business that cancer has become. Even our federal government is involved in the business of cancer: the U.S. Postal Service even sells a "Fund the Cure" stamp, purportedly to help "stamp out" breast cancer!

It is abnormal for fungi to live inside the human body. Fungi are ubiquitous in nature and are saprophytic. This means that they survive by ingesting dead or decaying material. Many fungi become parasitic once inside the human body. This fact may account for the dietary cravings that men and women have when suffering from internal yeast and fungal overgrowth. Parasites are alive and must eat. Fungal parasites must have sugar in order to thrive. So often we see people who eat very little, yet are extremely bloated, gaseous, and overweight. Most have numerous intestinal problems, including bloating, belching, gas, constipation, diarrhea, indigestion, or reflux. Ironically, most crave potatoes, pasta, sodas, bread, and sugar. *These are the very foods that fungi must have in order to thrive.* I have long contended that people who have fungal infections really can't control their cravings. They must keep the parasitic fungi fed or risk illness, themselves, as the fungi die!

Allow me to quote one sentence from a respected medical textbook: "That animals may be fattened on a predominantly carbohydrate diet demonstrates the ease of conversion of carbohydrate into fat." Yet again, nutritional myths of calorie counting or low-fat diets contributing to weight loss are exposed! Although this may be the case in some weight loss, it is certainly not the case in all. Ladies, it is very likely that if you have an internal fungal condition, the few foods you are eating are precisely the wrong ones. What about vegetarian diets? Remember, that fungi love tofu, breads, beans, and rice, but don't like meat. So many women that we counsel tell us that they eat a healthy vegetarian diet but feel miserable. I simply ask, "Healthy for whom?" Are *you* thriving, or is the fungus inside of you thriving?

You are probably tired of hearing me say, "Why hasn't any medical school or research organization resolved what seems so logical to you and me?" To solve this puzzle, simply travel 50 years back in time with me. Didn't four out of five doctors smoke Camels in 1948? Didn't we respect doctors enough to know that since they were medically trained, they *must* know what was necessary for optimum health?! Now this same profession is involved in litigation with the cigarette industry for something that their peers actively condoned a few decades ago! Was the past generation of physicians duped into believing that sucking on sugar-dipped tobacco leaves was really good for health; or did the tobacco industry literally buy their support from the American Medical Association?

Today, folks, it is likely that four out of five doctors prescribe antibiotics for their family members and their patients. No, doctors don't smoke any more; but you must understand that today medical schools receive millions of dollars in financial assistance not from the tobacco industry, but, rather, from the pharmaceutical industry. Where, then, are the medical institutions' loyalties today? Please think about this the next time you are handed a prescription following a brief medical exam. Is this really the best thing you can do for your medical condition, or was your doctor's medical training biased?

On the subject of yeast problems and women, David Holland, M. D., will give us his take on this interesting subject. Richard Mabray, M.D., a prominent gynecologist, has gained quite a reputation in medicine for his intense studies and research into the role of yeast and fungi in female health problems. You'll find Dr. Mabray's article very supportive of what you have really known all along: that yeast and fungi can cause debilitating medical symptoms.

When we finally comprehend the biases involved and the negative impact that many pharmaceutical drugs have had on our health, the field of medicine will begin to change. I'm certain that the power of an aroused public will have an impact on the very industry that *received* millions of dollars of very questionable grants and gifts, just as it did 50 years ago.

"Women and fungi" — far from the ideal date

David A. Holland, M.D.

> Study ties cases of vaginal thrush to baker's yeast! The yeast was apparently transferred from hand to vagina.
> -Medical Tribune, June 5, 1997

Statements researchers make are often more humorous than they are logical or scientific. The researchers responsible for the above headline may not have known of a study published 20 years earlier in the *Journal of the American Medical Association* (JAMA) where Mary Miles, M. D., et. al., discovered in 1977 that 100 percent of women with vaginal yeast had the same yeast isolated from their stools. They concluded that eradication of chronic yeast infections would be impossible without prior eradication of the gut yeast. In other words, the individuals in the study listed above probably contracted the vaginal yeast from *eating* the yeast bread! This has been questioned subsequently, however, because women can still become infested with vaginal yeast despite having negative stool cultures (C. C. Kibbler).

Why do we get these infections? I believe the answer lies in one's diet, or the *wrong* diet I should say. Again, this is just me

189

going out on a limb, but there is some rather compelling evidence that this may be true.

As you may recall, many fungi produce poisons called mycotoxins that can adversely affect their hosts (the human body, in this case). These mycotoxins suppress the immune system. They interfere with its normal function. In fact, we take advantage of this when we give kidney transplant recipients the mycotoxin called cyclosporine. Yes, this drug is a mycotoxin. Cyclosporine essentially shuts down our immune system so that the body will not reject the new kidney, which is basically a foreign object in the recipient's body. Our immune system is designed to reject foreign substances, but this reaction is not desirable in the case of a transplant. The negative aspect of immune suppression is that we are now left vulnerable to attack by *any* invading critter, namely fungal, bacterial, and viral organisms. If your immune system does not work, you will get sick!

Let's say that we are not taking the drug cyclosporine, which should be the case unless you just received a new kidney. How, then, can my immune system be suppressed by these fungal poisons, you might ask. The answer, again, may lie in your diet. Stored grains that become moldy are introduced either into the grain portion of your diet or your meats by way of cows and pigs being fed moldy grains. The FDA has established limits regarding the amount of *some* of the mycotoxins allowed in foods. Other potentially dangerous mycotoxins have had no limitations placed on them. Mycotoxins and molds are an insurmountable problem for farmers and can result in huge losses. For example, between 1977 and 1981 about one-third of the milled corn from the southeast U. S. contained levels of aflatoxin that were too high for human consumption (Mycotoxins, Economic and Health Risks. Task Force Report. No. 116. November 1989. Council for Agricultural Science and Technology – CAST). So where did that moldy corn go? It was diverted away from our table into cattle feed! So, even if we aren't consuming the contaminated grain directly, we may get chronic low levels in the fat of our meat (thus, trimming the fat may be useful for this reason and this only).

Some of these toxins, like aflatoxin, have been linked to cancers and atherosclerosis; but our interest for this chapter is in the role these toxins may play in female diseases. This is an interest of mine, as well. How many women do you hear of undergoing a hysterectomy due to fibroids? Or how many are getting breast biopsies because of a nodule they found? Or who doesn't know of someone who is having trouble getting pregnant, or even having trouble remaining pregnant? If a female is given high doses of the hormone estrogen, a number of atypical health events may take place including growth of the uterus and the breasts (could this *cause* cancer?). It would also be difficult for her to have a normal pregnancy because normal estrogen-progesterone ratios are needed by the body to both enable and maintain a pregnancy.

Let's say that you don't give her estrogen, but something that mimics it. A mycotoxin called zearalenone would fit that role. Interestingly, zearalenone is a mycotoxin found primarily in corn and corn-based products, such as cereal and corn meal, as well as in bananas world wide. It may also be a residue in the meat of cattle consuming contaminated corn (Mycotoxins. CAST.) Zearalenone is produced by a mold called *Fusarium graminearum*, which can invade and grow on corn in the field or in storage bins. Of interest is that zearalenone in cattle and swine has been associated with infertility and can interfere with fetal development, ovulation, conception, and viability of newborn animals. It can cause swelling of mammary glands and feminization of young male swine. The toxin mimics the effect of the hormone estrogen, and can have effects in concentrations as minute as one part per million!

What is being done to protect you against this toxin? The true answer is, "I don't know." While there are recommendations and enforced levels for a few mycotoxins, there are currently *no* limits or recommended levels of zearalenone placed on foods and grains for human consumption (Charles Wobshuk. Department of Botany and Plant Pathology. Purdue University). To have a zero-tolerance for these toxins would be cost-prohibitive; we just have to do the best we can.

As important as it is to uncover the fact that these problems exist in our food supply, of even greater importance is admitting they may be contributing to some chronic health problems. I would exercise caution with food choices. If you already have a weakened immune system or are chronically ill, then I'd change my diet and get that immune system working again. See the diet in the appendix for more information on this subject.

Maintaining
the delicate balance

C. R. Mabray, M.D.

Yeast infections and problems are so common that everyone, both healers and patients, know about them. And that's a problem! Most patients and nearly all physicians think of vaginal and vulvar itching, irritation, and discharge as all there is to a yeast "infection." Therefore, it simply does not compute that abnormal nail growth, scalding under the arms, acne, red rash around the mouth and nose, fatigue, joint pain, tendonitis, diarrhea, constipation, liver stress, etc. may all be symptoms of a yeast problem.

We have been brought up in a medical culture where we identify an offending germ or agent, find some drug to kill that offender, and then get "well." The problem is just not that simple. For many, if not most, the problem is an immune sensitivity to the yeast or a reaction to one of the scores of poisons or toxins that these yeasts are capable of producing. It is not always a simple infection. In fact, those with uncomplicated genital infections are the easiest to treat.

First, let me illustrate the immune aspect. We have poison ivy in our back yard from time to time. I can handle it with my bare hands and suffer no ill effect, whereas my son is so sensitive that he will suffer just being nearby while I cut and move the plant. He is "allergic" to poison ivy. In like manner, those having the most symptomatic and most treatment-resistant yeast problems are sensitive or "allergic" to the organism or to the toxins produced by the organism. Moreover, there is a close kin to other fungi, and folks most sensitive to candida yeasts almost always have heightened sensitivity to other yeasts, fungi, and molds. Thus, we must contend with one's total internal and external environment in order to get best treatment results. For example, if your house has been flooded and there is a fungal/mold growth in the walls or air-conditioning ducts or under the carpet, simply treating your yeast infection will neither restore nor maintain wellness. You must address the total load on your defense system.

Another significant problem with molds is their toxin production. Just the candida species, alone, has been demonstrated to have nearly 100 distinctly different powerful toxins (poisons) that have a specific impact on the human body. Some attack nervous tissue, some attack muscle, others attack connective tissues such as bone and joint tissue. Therefore, symptoms may vary dramatically depending upon the toxin produced, the target organ affected, and the integrity of our defense capabilities.

Bear in mind that "yeasts" are really not the problem. They are here on earth to be garbage recycling factories. If dead organisms were not recycled, the earth would cease to be habitable – dead things would just pile up to the moon. Converting dead organisms to a useable form requires the powerful chemical secretions of yeasts, mold, fungi, and bacteria which are capable of transforming once-living organisms into "dirt."

The process of life may begin again through the miracle of photosynthesis, which is the basis of our whole food chain and existence. These toxins must be powerful to do their job. They are meant to be a blessing. It is only when the system gets out of balance inside our bodies through stress, antibiotic exposure, high-sugar diet, injury, chemical exposure, etc. that the toxins become our enemy rather than our friend.

In summary, yeast problems vary from easy and straightforward to complex and convoluted. Symptoms may occur because of infection, sensitivity (allergy), toxin exposure, or some combination. These symptoms seldom exist without an imbalance in your personal eco-life-health system.

The successful defeat of symptoms may involve simple changes of lifestyle and environment, or may respond only to drastic adjustments, plus supplements, plus allergy management, plus medication. In either case, be prepared to take control of your own life and health – that's the only way it works well!

Chapter Ten

Fungi and Pain

Fungi's ability to cause pain

Doug A. Kaufmann

According to the book, *Alternative Medicine,*[*] chronic pain has become the United States' most common health disorder, affecting nearly one in three Americans and costing nearly 40 billion dollars a year in bills and lost wages. With another one in three of us suffering from heart disease and another one in three suffering from cancer, well, you get the picture. That which isn't killing us is hurting us!

My own back pain became so unbearable in my early 20s that my roommates jokingly rigged up a pulley over my bed to assist me in getting up each morning. There were actually days I wished it were functional, because I would have used it! Twenty-eight years later, although I have had intermittent flare-ups on rare occasions, my back pain is gone. Most importantly, I know exactly how to exacerbate this horrible pain. Why is that so important? Well, if you know how to provoke pain, then you also know how to subdue it. Ironically, when I consume too much sugar, my back pain is upon me like white on rice. If I dare sleep in the wrong position or lift anything the day after a sugar binge, you can bet money that I'll be out of commission for a few days. Logic might dictate, therefore, that as the bread-winner in my family, I avoid sugar and, therefore, avoid lost time at work. The combination of being self-employed and breadwinner is especially tough because when I don't work, we don't eat. As a quick learner, I carefully choose my down time. I happen to love mom's fudge at Christmas time. I take two weeks off at year's end for a totally different reason than most people: recuperation!

Pain is so common that ten years ago a prominent headache specialist wrote a book educating physicians on the proper meth-ods of encoding insurance forms for payment when dealing with headaches. Entitled *Headache Classification System, A Diagnostic Code Manual*, this book contains 376 pages. Mind you, this is only headache pain! Just imagine the diagnostic book for back pain! I had a chiropractic friend who had a giant book which listed the causes of subluxation (a dislocation of a joint, so that the bone ends are misaligned but still in contact) and general back pain. Lifting the book was listed on page 945! The point is, there are as many causes of pain as there are people with pain. Neither of these books on back or headache pain listed sugar or fungus as etiologic factors, but they sure do pro-voke my back pain! Sugars feed parasitic fungus. Like many things in medicine, these books prove that the simplest con-cepts are often the last to be accepted.

Those who suffer from pain tend to be their own best doctors. I have always believed that the best orthopedic physicians in the world would be those who suffered from pain. You can bet that these physicians have employed techniques in their practices additional to what medical school taught them. Life experiences often provide better lessons than books.

You know that I believe that fungus, either acting alone or in unison with its metabolites, causes nearly every malady known to man. The two leading causes of death in the United States are heart disease and cancer. There is reason to believe that we remain ignorant as to why these diseases are killing so many because the medical profession has not been properly educated in the field of mycology, the study of fungi.

We have expounded upon both the physical symptoms caused by fungi and the impact of fungi on the brain and nervous system. As you may recall, several respected scientific authors have concluded that fungi, once inside the human body, are known to disseminate. This spreading of fungi can lead to tissue impregnation and affect tissues and organs far from the original portal of entry. The portal of entry can be respiratory, via inhalation of spores, can be the skin, via puncture or transdermal entrance, can be ingesting it through what we eat, or can be the end result of sexual contact with a person that has a localized fungal disease in the genitalia.

Once parasitic fungi have found a new host, numerous symptoms and diseases can be initiated but not always immediately. I happen to believe that in most healthy individuals, although dissemination can occur quickly, pain and suffering caused by these fungi may take decades. For this reason, do not ever underestimate the fact that your pain may be linked with a slow growing, insidious pathogen. If this were the case, what preexisting conditions would have led to the subjective symptoms, called pain, that you now suffer from?

As I mentioned earlier, my pain is directly linked with sugar. Ironically, the pain does not exacerbate upon eating sugar on each occurrence. I might not experience any pain associated with eating a bowl of ice cream. If I stop there, I'm fine! I still feel, however, that I have this underlying addiction to sugar. So the harmless bowl of ice cream becomes a bowl of pasta the following evening, followed by a dessert that I rarely eat. Soon, I'm finding it impossible to avoid potatoes, excessive fruits, and even chocolate. Before this addiction has ended, you can bet that during my daily routine I'll twist the wrong way and, BINGO, the pain begins. The difference in your pain and my pain is that, during the past 25 years, I've been able to trace mine directly to increased carbohydrate consumption. It is my contention that nine in ten of you would be able to discover the etiology of your pain given enough time and a sincere interest in the root cause, thereby leading to recovery. After reading this chapter, you may want to take steps enabling you to not only discover the roots of your pain, but also to eliminate it!

*Burton Goldberg Group. *Alternative Medicine:The definitive guide.* 1995. Future Medicine Publishing, Inc. Fife, Washington.

Fibromyalgia and Chronic Fatigue Syndrome

David A. Holland, M.D.

In this section, I will discuss what we believe, based on clinical observation, to be the cause of FM and CFS. Although the two conditions constitute two, separate disorders, they share so many symptoms that it only makes sense to consider them together.

Definitions

Fibromyalgia (FM) — a disorder of *unknown etiology* character-ized by, among many other symptoms, fatigue, musculoskel-etal pain, and muscle stiffness (*Harrison's Principles of Internal Medicine*. 12ᵗʰ Ed. 1991.)

Chronic fatigue syndrome (CFS) — also of *unknown etiology*, is currently diagnosed by the occurrence of:

➢New onset fatigue of greater than six month duration with a 50 percent decrease in normal activity.

➢No other medical or psychiatric conditions that could ex-plain the symptoms.

➢and six to eight of the symptoms and at least two physical

signs described below (all eight symptoms would make identi-
fication of signs unnecessary).

Symptoms: low-grade fever, sore throat, painful lymph node
swelling, generalized muscle weakness, muscle aches, headaches,
migratory joint aches, and sleep disturbances

Signs: body temperature of 37.5–38.6 degrees C, pharyngitis,
or palpable cervical or axillary lymph node swelling
(*Griffith's Five-Minute Clinical Consultant.* 1991.)

You may have detemined that you have CFS just from reading
the list! Never mind technicalities; these are used for diagnostic
purposes. If you have been diagnosed with FM or CFS, then
once you get past the medical jargon, all you really care about is
that you feel BAD and you want to know what you can do to
feel GOOD!

I looked up CFS on the internet and came up with more than
100,000 sites to search through. I quit after reviewing a hundred or so, because it soon became clear that no one was coming up with any definitive answers regarding these elusive disorders, despite the large number of unproven theories.

Myalgic encephalomyelitis, a term introduced in 1957 in the
United Kingdom, is what we know today in the United States

as chronic fatigue syndrome (Scand, J. Work Environment Health. Suppl. 23. 1997. 3:17-34). The timing of the appearance of this "disorder" is interesting in that antibiotic use was becoming more prevalent at the time, having recently been introduced as the new "magic bullet" for bacterial infections. One might wonder if the timing is more than coincidence, since it is well known that antibiotic use is a risk factor for yeast and fungal overgrowth (Kibbler, C. C. *Principles and Practice of Clinical Mycology.* 1996. Pg. 9).

Is there any proof that fungi and yeast cause FM or CFS? None, directly, that I came across. However, one must examine cause and effect and consider what treatments have worked to retrospectively diagnose what must have been the cause. I have seen, time and time again, clients initiate an anti-fungal/anti-mycotoxin diet and take anti-fungal medications in an attempt to rid themselves of their fatigue, only to have complete and long term success and recovery. *If the successful treatment was antifungal, then the cause was fungal!*

It has been said that no amount of negative studies can offset one single positive clinical observation. In addition, it would be difficult to isolate the causative fungus in any situation to prove a link, since "*dissemination of yeasts is unlikely to be recognized because they are rarely identified ... in the routine labora-*

tory." (Kibbler, C. C.) Our medical laboratories are simply not adept at routinely isolating fungi from human tissue or fluid samples.

I did come across one study (*Medical Hypotheses.* June, 1995. 44[6]:507-515) describing the fact that patients with "chronic candidiasis syndrome" shared many of the same symptoms as those with CFS. It also mentioned that patients with CFS had improvement in their symptoms after taking oral anti-fungal medication. Lastly, the study acknowledged the fact that patients with *Candida* overgrowth (as in chronic mucocutaneous candidiasis) had suppression in their cellular immunity, a finding also seen in CFS patients. Without an intact cellular immune system, one is susceptible to reactivation of such viral infections as shingles, herpes zoster, and Epstein-Barr virus (EBV). Thus, in cases of CFS that were suspected to be *caused* by EBV, one can now see that the true initiating factor of the fatigue was the fungal overgrowth, or more rightly so, the factor *that caused the fungal overgrowth*, whether it be antibiotics, birth control pills, etc.

A chapter in *Mycotoxins: Economic and Health Risks* (CAST Task Force Report No. 116. November, 1989. Phone 515-

292-2125) discusses in extensive detail the means by which several common mycotoxins impair the immune system. Without an immune system that works, it is inevitable that one will remain chronically ill and susceptible to secondary viral, fungal, and bacterial infections as long as one is exposed to the source of these toxins. Remember, fungi are ubiquitous – they are every where! Again, these toxins may be antibiotics or other mycotoxins that can be found in moldy grains or in moldy-grain-fed animals.

Thus, once again, we have two conditions that have *enormous* economic impact in terms of lost productivity, diagnosis, and treatment, and, yet, no real answers in the medical field to offer these patients. The huge success with the approaches mentioned above should at the very least behoove the medical community to take a closer look into these so called "alternative" approaches to treatment. This is especially true given the fact that prescriptive medicines like hormones and antibiotics used to treat patients may, in fact, be contributing to the cause of FM and CFS! Having seen the anti-fungal/anti-mycotoxin diet approach work, I am thoroughly convinced that in most, if not all, cases, there is a fungal etiology to FM and CFS.

Craniosacral Manipulation Therapy

What to do if your pain fails to respond to antifungal treatments or a change in diet

Richard Becker, D.O.

As an osteopathic physician, I have come to respect the body's ability to heal itself when given the opportunity to do so. The nerves that control our organs and systemic reactions all come through and around our spine. If the spine is not free to engage full range of motion, pain often ensues. Pain is not the only down side to this condition. A nervous reflex can inhibit healthy organ function which, in turn, can result in disease.

Craniosacral manipulation therapy (CMT) is a form of hands-on physical medicine aimed at correcting the spinal misalignments. Manual manipulation of basic physiologic processes can restore the integrity of the spinal pathways thereby relieving the tissues of pressure they have assumed with the misalignment. As you know, tissues of the body have circulation, otherwise stagnation will occur. The heart consistently pumps blood through the blood vessels. Cerebrospinal fluid (CSF), however, does not have a pumping mechanism to cause circulation. So, just how does the CSF circulate? One chamber of the brain houses the choroid plexus. This plexus actually

213

produces CSF. Tiny, thin layers surrounding the brain and the spinal chord called *meninges* contain small, finger-like projections called *arachnoid villae*. These tiny structures reabsorb CSF. Unlike the constant pumping of the heart to circulate blood, these two CSF processes do not occur simultaneously. Rather, they ebb and flow like the waves in the ocean. In doing so, a pressure wave is created throughout the human body. Skilled osteopathic physicians can literally feel this pulse inside the body and determine blockages. When the spine or internal organs are damaged or diseased, the pressure wave is inhibited. A small amount of pressure (5 – 10 grams), succinctly placed, will completely stop this vital flow of cerebrospinal fluid. By holding the spinal column in a corrupted position, away from the muscle and connective tissue tension, there will be neurologic influences stimulated, thereby restoring proper alignment and active cranial rhythm. Proper blood flow, essential to health, is also restored.

Sounds great, doesn't it? Best of all, it really works! It takes many years of training to perfect this method of treatment, and each therapeutic session requires 30 to 60 minutes to perform. As Doug has told you before, most physicians see 40 to 50 patients daily and could not, therefore, perform such treatments for their patients. This is unfortunate for both the practitioner as well as their patients.

Craniosacral therapy has been proven to help a wide variety of disorders, including arthritis, chronic joint pain, traumatic injuries, bursitis, tendonitis, and a variety of internal organ conditions previously thought to respond only to medications. If you are suffering from ongoing pain, or would simply like to "jump start" your nerves and muscles to good health, consider craniosacral manipulation therapy. It is safe, natural, and, most importantly, it's effective!

Prolotherapy

by Doug A. Kaufmann

Pastor Peter did not survive his deadly cancer. After his death, his close friend, Dr. Ross Hauser, and I stayed in touch with one another, communicating over the fax machine several times weekly. Dr. Hauser is a highly specialized pain therapist called a physiatrist (pron. *fizzy-a-trist*). Such credentials require a graduate medical degree and then an additional four years of residency. There are approximately 5,000 physiatrists in the United States, but only one Ross Hauser. Ross puts the "gentle" in gentleman. His wife, Marion, is the perfect addition to his hectic life. Get these two alone and you'll fully comprehend the opening admonition in his book that you need to lighten up and laugh more often!

Like Dr. Richard Becker, Dr. Hauser's therapy requires the highly skilled brain and hands of a physician. Don't try this on yourself at home! Dr. Hauser performs a therapy called "prolotherapy." This therapy stimulates the areas of pain by inducing an inflammation at the site of pain or injury. This is accomplished by using very thin-gauged needles to direct the natural medicines in the syringe to a specific site. A small amount of the formula is then injected, and several sites surrounding the injury are also injected. It is not uncommon to have Dr. Hauser inject 20 to 50 times during one visit. Since the injections contain a numbing ingredient, this is not as painful as it sounds. Several visits are often required to terminate the pain, but many people claim to have significant relief following the initial visit. As is the case with Dr. Becker's craniosacral therapy, a variety of pain conditions, including arthritis, back pain, migraine head-aches, fibromyalgia, sports injuries, TMJ, herniated discs, and sciatica have all responded favorably to prolotherapy.

Dr. Ross and Marion reduced their knowledge to book form a few years ago. This remarkable book, entitled *Prolo Your Pain Away*, has been so successful that a sequel is forthcoming. The new book will expound on sports injuries and the ability of prolotherapy to cure these.

Yes, I said *cure*. Why is it that this has become the "four letter word" in clinical medicine? Simply put, the Wall Street beau-ties of conventional medicine (i.e., pharmaceutical drugs) don't cure anything but the overgrowth of bacteria – and even that returns! They certainly can't cure depression, Alzheimer's dis-ease, or even pain! Despite this, their sales figure are impressive, a clear indication that we prefer adding annuities to the phar-maceutical coffers over investigating breakthrough technolo-gies like prolotherapy.

If you do decide to investigate, don't be surprised if your orthopedic physician gives you the cold shoulder. Do you remember the name that is used for anything that competes with organized medicine? The technology is called "quackery," while the therapists are called "quacks." Based on everything I've learned about honesty and integrity in medicine, I am left wondering who the real "quacks" are!

I have witnessed Dr. Hauser at work on several occasions and have had the opportunity to interview the patients he has performed prolotherapy on. All of the patients I witnessed receiving prolo are thankful and thrilled with the therapy. If your pain is chronic and unrelenting, please consider a hands-on approach – not hands-on a prescription pad, but hands on you!

Chapter 11

Doug Kaufmann's
Antifungal Program

featuring the

Initial Phase and
InterPhase diets

The Program

An explanation
of fungal therapy

Localized or systemic (throughout the body) mycoses (fungi) are not rare. As a matter of fact, they were once commonly and openly referred to within scientific literature as quite common. However, the popularity of bacteria and viruses eventually overshadowed the field of mycology (the study of fungi) and fungi were pushed to the side. Only recently, with accelerated use of chemotherapy, antibiotics, and steroid therapy, have fungi begun to emerge as a serious cause of human illness. This is because immunosuppressed (weak immune system) or hypoimmune hosts (people) are prey to these opportunistic yeasts. "Opportunistic" means that weakened immunity gives opportunity for a fungal infection to thrive. What we do not seem to realize is that *all* of us exposed to antibiotics, steroids, birth control pills, and polluted air, food, and water are likely immunocompromised to some degree.

Fungi can be treated with the use of pharmaceutical drugs or natural remedies depending upon the severity of the infection. Although both remedies seem to work well, drugs sometimes work more quickly. Depending on the type of fungi, a physician may prescribe Nystatin, Lamisil, Nizoral, Diflucan, or

Sporanox. Each of these is a prescriptive medicine and each has published side effects.

If you choose to address a fungal problem with natural remedies, you have literally hundreds of options. Some of the most common are listed in this chapter.

Starve the fungi

Our Initial Phase Diet (IPD) defines our approach to ridding the body of fungal organisms by starving them. Scientific literature has long referred to dietary patterns that allow fungi to proliferate. We know, for example, that sugar fuels the growth pattern for yeast and fungi. Considering that each American man, woman, and child consumes approximately 130 pounds of sugar annually, it is not surprising that fungi are so difficult to control once they become activated within the human body. Most of us think that the sugars we consume are limited to candy and soda pop. Although our average consumption of soda in America averages 50 gallons yearly per person, our sugar intake is certainly not limited to this type of sugar. Avoiding carbohydrates is also important.

The *Bantam Medical Dictionary* defines carbohydrates as:

any one of a large group of compounds including the sugars and starch that contain carbon, hydrogen, and oxygen. Carbohydrates are manufactured by plants and obtained by animals and man from the diet, being one of the three main constituents of food, besides protein and fat. All carbohydrates are eventually broken down in the body to the simple sugar, glucose, which can then take part in energy-producing metabolic processes.

Carbohydrates are fuel for the body. This fuel is generated by the body's breakdown of certain carbohydrates into sugars. Yet sugar also feeds fungi. Ironically, most of the clients who have fungal disorders consume too much sugar and are exhausted! The right type of carbohydrate in a non-toxic individual will supply energy, however the wrong type of carbohydrate in a fungally-toxic individual actually suppresses energy.

Not only is it important to starve yeasts and fungi, but it is important to avoid and minimize the potent toxins they produce. Vegetables absorb fungal poisons called mycotoxins, carry them out of the body, and inhibit their toxicity. Carotenoids are good chemicals found in vegetables, including xanthophylls, lutein, and lycopene. In one study, carotenoids were found to block the cancer-causing ability of aflatoxin B1 and T2 mycotoxins in experimental animals. Aflatoxin is produced by the mold *Aspergillus* and T2 is made from *Fusarium* mold; both are well known cancer-causing poisons. It has been speculated that the vegetable carotenoids are the very reason vegetables protect against cancer.

Get and Keep the Bowels Moving

It is imperative that, as you kill fungi, they are eliminated from the body. This is a job for the bowels, and too often it is a job poorly done. Non-digestible fiber assists the body in ridding impacted wastes and aids in bowel regularity. The term "non-digestible" means that what goes in must come out, and it will in due time. We specifically recommend psyllium hulls or slippery elm as good sources of this type of fiber. These are available in health food stores and we have found that the powder form is best. Both of these products tend to work best when taken either at the hour of sleep (one tablespoon mixed into water) or divided throughout the day (one heaping teaspoon in water twice daily). It is important to drink plenty of water when taking these forms of fiber. Bottled, spring water, or reverse osmosis water is best. Bulk fibers, such as psyllium hulls and slippery elm, should be used at the discretion of your physician if you have had bowel surgery or a history of intestinal blockage.

If you are constipated and the fiber does not regulate you, you might try cascara sagrada, also obtainable from a health food store. Cascara sagrada stimulates peristalsis (moving of the intestines) and should not be taken for long periods of time. Also note that magnesium deficiency can be another cause of constipation.

227

Repair Oxidative Damage

Free radical molecules are harmful chemicals which can contribute to many symptoms. Skin collagen damage related to free radical injury can be determined with two simple tests.

Do you have a vertical crease in your earlobe? Interestingly, you may be at an increased risk of heart and circulatory damage.

With your hand and arm flat on a table, lift the skin on the back of your hand for a few seconds. Does it snap back when released or does it return to its original dimension slowly? If it returns slowly, this is yet another indication of free radical tissue damage and/or dehydration. If this process occurs on the skin, just imagine what must be going on inside your body!

Proanthocyanidins (PC) are a class of free radical scavengers. You may have heard of two of these PCs, Pycnogenol and grape seed extract. Any health food store has these supplements. At present there is no lab method for determining percentages of OPC (oligomeric proanthocyanidins). Additionally, grape seeds have galic esters, making them more desirable. The usual dosage is approximately one milligram per pound of body weight per day in two or three doses, but it is safe to begin with a larger "loading" dose.

Kill the Fungus

Only a physician can prescribe a pharmaceutical drug. You, however, may elect to try the following remedies, each of which has antifungal properties. These are available in health food stores, health or organic sections of grocery stores, or nutritionally-oriented pharmacies.

1. Olive leaf extracts (OLE) are antimicrobial agents. Independent lab tests have demonstrated the ability of OLE to eradicate pathogens (any organism capable of causing a disease). OLE contains oleuropein and other active phytochemicals which are responsible for their antimicrobial abilities.

2. Caprylic acid is a fatty acid derived from coconut oil. It has potent antifungal properties.

3. Pau d'arco is another good antifungal that is either taken in tea form or in capsules. It comes from the bark of the pau d'arco tree which contains the fungicides. Despite very high humidity in the rain forest, the pau d'arco tree does not grow mold or mildew on its bark.

4. FORMULA SF722 is actually a brand name (Thorpe Research) for undecalynic acid. Derived from the oil of caster beans, this is another good, antifungal product.

5. Malic acid is derived from apple cider vinegar and has strong, antifungal properties. This can be diluted with water or mixed with fresh-squeezed juice.

6. Garlic is one of the most well published antifungals in the world. One of the phyto (plant) enzymes in garlic, **allicin**, is well documented as having anti-microbial properties not limited to the eradication of fungi. It appears viruses and bacteria are also neutralized by garlic. Many supplement companies sell garlic, but since allicin is best used synergistically with other enzymes contained in the garlic, it is best (and most cost effective) to squeeze a clove into your fresh carrot juice.

7. Carrot juice contains many important properties, not the least of which inhibits fungal proliferation. A 1988 study in *The Journal of Microbiology* implicated carrot as a good, fungus fighter. Again, although the pulp is very important in the carrot, juicing gives your blood stream immediately-available nutrition and gives your digestive juices a break from digesting whole foods.

8. Tea tree oil, available in health food stores, seems to work quickly and effectively on local skin fungal problems. Time may prove that anything that survives the germination process in soil has antifungal properties. Fungus would have taken over the world if it were not for antifungal properties in soil. Certain antifungal drugs that we recommend, including nystatin, are actually derived from fungi that live in the soil. It is important, therefore, to remember the value of organically grown fresh vegetables. Not only are they nutritious, but they may also be antifungal remedies.

9. Grapefruit see extract (GSE) is more effective at killing yeast than chlorine bleach, colloidal silver, tea tree oil and io-dine (*GSE Report*, Volume 1, Issue 1, pg. 6).

I. The Initial Phase Diet
(formerly the Phase One Diet)

Food Groups	Foods ALLOWED on the diet	Foods EXCLUDED from the diet
1. Sugar	None[a]	All sugars excluded
2. Artificial and herbal sweeteners	Stevia, Stevia Plus	Aspartame, saccharin
3. Fruit	Green apples, berries, avocados, grapefruit, lemons, limes	All others, including fruit juices
4. Meat	Virtually all meats, including fish, poultry and beef[b]	Breaded meats
5. Eggs	Yes, all types allowed	Avoid egg substitutes
6. Dairy[c]	Yogurt (especially goat yogurt) cream cheese, unsweetened whipping cream, sour cream made from real cream, butter	All others, including margarine and any of the butter substitutes
7. Vegetables	Most fresh, unblemished vegetables and freshly made vegetable juice[d]	Potatoes and legumes (beans and peas)
8. Beverages	Bottled/filtered water; non-fruity, herb teas; Stevia-sweetened, fresh lemonade or lime-ade	Coffee and tea (including decaf) and regular/diet sodas
9. Grains	Zero grains allowed	Pasta, rice, corn, wheat, quinoa, amaranth, millet, buckwheat, oats and barley
10. Yeast Products	No yeast allowed	All are all *excluded*, as are bread, mushrooms, pastries and alcohol
11. Vinegars	Unpasteurized, apple cider vinegar and black olives not aged in vinegar	Pickles, salad dressings[e] green olives, soy sauce
12. Oils	Olive, grape seed, flax seed etc. (use cold pressed when available)	Partially-hydrogenated ("trans") oils, corn and peanut oil
13. Nuts	Raw nuts, including pecans, almonds, walnuts, cashews, pumpkin seeds	Peanuts (and all peanut products) and pistachios are excluded.

(p. 232)

II. InterPhase

(formerly the Phase Two Diet)

Food Groups	Foods ALLOWED in the diet	Foods EXCLUDED from the diet
1. Sugar		
2. Artificial and herbal sweeteners	*Same as Initial Phase Diet* for food groups number one through six.	
3. Fruit		
4. Meat		
5. Eggs		
6. Dairy[c]		
7. Vegetables	Fresh, unblemished vegetables and freshly made vegetable juice,[d] *yams, legumes (beans and peas)*	Potatoes
8. Beverages	Bottled/filtered water; non-fruity, herb teas; Stevia-sweetened, fresh lemonade or lime-ade	Coffee and tea (including decaf) and sodas (diet sodas also excluded)
9. Grains	*Oats (oatmeal), brown rice, quinoa, amaranth, millet, buckwheat, barley, flour tortillas, sourdough bread (in moderation)*	Corn and yeast breads
10. Yeast Products		
11. Vinegars	**Same as *Initial Phase Diet* for food groups number ten through thirteen.**	
12. Oils		
13. Nuts		

Notes for Initial Phase and InterPhase

a. Honey may be used sparingly as a sweetner if needed.

b. Farm-raised meat and fish are corn-fed, so they should be kept to a minimum. Grass-fed beef is ideal, followed by organic meats to which antibiotic exposure has been minimized.

c. Dairy products are better if from range-fed cattle and animals not injected with antibiotics, hormones or steroids, nor fed with silo stored grains. Good products include Brown Cow, Monarch Hills and Redwood Hills. Whipping cream is liquid, unsweetened, heavy cream.

d. Organically grown vegetables are preferred.

e. Excluded because many of them are fermented products.

Additional facts about food

Many of the pre-packaged foods you find on store shelves contain unhealthy ingredients. The following lists should assist you in spotting those ingredients that should be *excluded* when following the Initial Phase and InterPhase diets. Investigate and read all labels, please.

Dairy

cow's milk
casein
caseinate
sodium caseinate

whey
lactalbumin
lactalbumin phosphate
buttermilk (solids included)

The food industry also produces "Non-Dairy" or "Dairy Free" products; these should also be *excluded* from the diet.

Sugar

lactose (milk/dairy)
sucrose
glucose
maltodextrose
maltose
dextrose

fructose
corn syrup
corn syrup solids
honey
maple syrup

We should note that honey can be eaten occasionally, albeit sparingly, because it does possess antifungal properties that the other sugars do not. Artificials sweeters are off-limits. These include Nutra-Sweet (aspartame), and saccharine.

(continued on following page)

Vinegars

catsup/ketchup	pickles	green olives
mustard	pickled peppers	horscradish
BBQ sauce	hot sauce	dips
soy sauce	salad dressings	mayonnaise
Worcestershire sauce		

The above items have been fermented, and should be *excluded*.

Yeast

Hydrolyzed yeast is an additive in many products such as canned and powdered soups and frozen dinners. *Look for it!*

Good Food Choices
Vegetables

alfalfa sprouts
artichoke, Chinese
asparagus
bamboo sprouts
banana peppers
Bavarian endive
  (escarole, chicory escarole)
bean sprouts
beets
beet greens
bell pepper (sweet green & red)
Brussels sprouts
cabbages —
  bok choy
  broccoli
  cabbage kraut
  cauliflower
  celery cabbage
  Chinese cabbage
  collard greens
  head (green, red)
  kale
  kohlrabi
  savoy
capers, without vinegar
cardoon
carrots
chayte
celery
celeriac (celery root, knob celery)

dandelion greens
dulse
eggplant
fennel (finoccio)
garden cress
garlic
kelp (seaweed)
Lamb's Quarters
leeks
lettuces —
  butterhead
  bib
  Boston
  celtuce (stem)
  iceberg (crisp head)
  loose-leaf
  Lamb's
  matchless
  Oakleaf (green bronze)
  Prizehead
  salad bowl
  red leaf chicory
  argula
  Romaine (cos)
roguette
rutabaga
onion
okra
parsnip
pumpkin

Vegetables (continued)

sea kale
shallots
spinach
squashes —
    acorn
    alligator
    banana
    Boston marrow
    bush
    buttercup
    butternut
    Caserta
    cheese
    cocozelle
    Connecticut field
    cushaw
    Delicious
    Golden Nugget
    hubbard varieties
    mammoth
    Mirliton
    pumpkin
    quaker pie
    Queensland
    straightneck
    Table Queen
    Turbin Virginian
    whitebush scallop
    zucchini
Swiss chard

tomatillo
tomatoes, all kinds
turnip greens
upland cress
water cress
Whitloff chicory (Belgian or
                French endive)
yucca

Miscellaneous

agar-agar
aloe vera
carrageen (Irish moss)
pepino (melon pear)
rhubarb

Good Food Choices
Meats

beef
  bologna
  liver
  sausage
  milk product: plain yogurt
buffalo
goat (kid) — milk, cheese
lamb
pork —
  ham
  sausage, etc.
poultry —
  chicken & chicken eggs
  dove
  duck & duck eggs
  goose & goose eggs
  guinea hen
  pea fowl
  pheasant
  prairie chicken
  quail
  turkey & turkey eggs
seafood —
crustaceans:
  cray fish
  Dungeness crab
  lobster
  shrimp (prawns)
  snow crab

seafood (cont.) —
  octopus
  scallop
  snail
  squid
fresh water fish:
  beluga
  carp
  catfish
  caviar (roe)
  crapapie (crappie)
  pickerel
  salmon
  smelt
  sturgeon
  trout, all species
  perch
  whitefish
  yellow bass
salt water fish:
  albacore tuna
  anchovy
  bluefish
  cod (scrod)
  flounder
  haddock
  halibut
  Mahi-Mahi
  ocean catfish

Meats (continued)

sea food (cont.) —
    salt water fish, continued:
        red snapper
        sea bass
        sea herring
        swordfish
        tuna
veal
venison (deer)

Miscellaneous (The following are not recommended for frequent consumption due to processing and fermentation. Processing can include starch fillers and sugars.)

bologna
frankfurters
sausage
salami

Good food choices
Herbs and spices

allspice
althea root (tea)
angelica
anise
apple mint
balm
basil
bergamot
boneset (tea)
borage
burdock root (tea)
burnet (cucumber flavor)
caraway
cardamom
cassia
celery seed
chamomile (tea)
chervil
chicory (in tea)
chive
cilantro/coriander
clove
comfrey (tea)
cumin
dittany
dry mustard
East Indian arrowroot
fenugreek
ginger
ginseng (tea)

hibiscus, roselle (tea)
horehound
horseradish
lavender
lemon balm (Melissa)
licorice
lovage
mace
marjoram
menthol
mint
nutmeg
oregano
paprika/paprica
parsley
peppercorns (black, white)
peppermint
pimento
rosemary
saffron
sage
savory
sorrel (dock)
spearmint
tarragon
thyme
turmeric

Miscellaneous
sea salt

Appendices

Doug and Dr. Dave answer some

Frequently Asked Questions

Will I be on this diet forever?

No, you will not be on the IPD forever, unless you choose to do so. Our Initial Phase Diet (IPD) presents a shock to most people. One consolation for you is knowing that everyone on the staff here at Mediatrition has been on the diet. We're not asking you to do something we have not done ourselves.

Not much is known about fungal diseases, because in the 1970s the Center for Disease Control (CDC) decided that fungal diseases were not classified as "notifiable diseases." This means that doctors are not required to report these conditions to regulatory agencies. Hence, a dietary program has never been officially established. The IPD was born out of our understanding of which foods fed living fungi and which did not. In essence, we are asking you to take the next 14 days to see if you feel better. If you do feel better, this may be due to one of two things: either you have literally starved the living parasitic fungi, microorganisms that must feed on carbohydrates, or you have avoided specific food that you are allergic to. In either case, we will begin experimenting with the reintroduction phase of this program, thereby establishing threshold levels of tolerance to certain carbohydrates and food. Do not be fooled into believing that a 14-day diet will "cure" your fungus problems. We are using this next 14 days to establish whether or not you have a fungal problem and the extent or severity of your condition.

Won't eating eggs and nuts raise my cholesterol?

A great question and one that I asked myself twenty years ago. My experience has been quite the opposite! Blood fats actually reduce while following the IPD. As a matter of fact, fungi produce sterol (cholesterol) and triglycerides. By ridding the body of fungus, blood fats diminish. Recently, studies have confirmed that eggs do not necessarily raise cholesterol after all, and that eating nuts (not peanuts) can even decrease your risk of heart disease by up to 50%!

The general public has been frightened by fat in their diet and often beneficial fats are avoided. Less than one percent of the population actually suffers from a condition where the body cannot handle dietary cholesterol. If you have this rare genetic condition, please speak with your doctor prior to initiating the IPD. Keep in mind that each of us is biochemically unique. The IPD may work wonderfully for one person. It may not work for everyone.

Isn't fat bad for you? Won't I gain weight on the IPD?

There are good fats and bad fats. Eating bad fats is bad, eating good fats is not bad. What are bad fats? Well, margarine and vegetable oils used over and over for deep-frying in restaurants are examples of bad fats. Avocados, raw nuts (except peanuts), eggs, and organic, range-fed meats are all fine. We should, however, note a disclaimer on meats: meat from cattle fed moldy grains (i.e., corn or wheat) is not good. Be careful of restaurant and grocery store meats. The fats of these meats may contain mycotoxins from cattle eating moldy grains.

Have you heard anywhere that meat can cause heart disease and cancer? Mycotoxins are thought to be the reason. Not because of the meat, but because of the dangers associated with our consumption of cattle fed moldy grains. Argentineans consume more beef than any one in the world, yet they have no heart disease or cancer as a result of this. Why? They let their cattle graze in the open fields instead of feeding them moldy grain from silos like we do in the United States.

How will I feel during the program?

Always remember the adage, "No pain, no gain." As we starve yeast and fungi, a phenomenon called "Herxheimer's reaction" may occur. In the 1930s, German dermatologist Dr. Carl Herxheimer first described the body's reaction to the massive killing of microorganisms and the resulting sudden load of toxins released into the blood stream. Also known as "die off," these reactions are typically characterized by flu-like symptoms, chills, aches, and sometimes a low grade fever. It is not rare to suffer from a worsening of the very symptoms you originally experienced. Thirty to forty percent of our clients notice "die off" reactions. This reaction is often a good sign as it verifies that you have been harboring these fungi for quite some time and you have now begun to eradicate them. Like any living thing, they don't like to die! Also, recall that the skin is the largest organ in your body, so it is not rare to see outbreaks or worsening of rashes as the body begins to "clean house." Taking Essiac tea two or three times daily can significantly lessen the Herxheimer's reaction.

How will you know that this is not a reaction to something you are taking? If you are reacting to something that you have just started, you will feel worse and worse. Not so if you are experiencing a "die off" reaction. Within a few days you will feel much better even though you continue taking the supplement. In our experience, the longer the "die off" reaction, the more severe the fungal problem; however, this is not always predictable.

How can I prove that I have a fungal problem?

There are fairly accurate blood tests that detect the presence of antibodoes to fungi within the blood stream. One problem with blood tests is that they can detect a past exposure to fungi; however, they are sometimes inaccurate in picking up present symptoms caused by fungi. Also, by the time these test results are returned to our office, often the client following our program already feels much improvement, thereby ruling out the necessity for the expensive tests. We feel that the best way to confirm that a fungal problem exists is to begin our program and if, within a few days to a few weeks you feel much better, that might be all the confirmation you needed! Also, your response to a fungal questionnaire would be another clue. Often a good medical history tends to support or rule out suspicions of fungal growth. (Note: please see our questionnaire, *Your Fungal Quotient*, for more answers to this question. The questionnaire is located in the appendix.)

Is a fungal disorder a "forever" disorder, or can fungi be successfully eradicated?

This is one of the good questions that we are asked every day. Although our IPD and program will not have to be followed forever, please keep in mind that fungi cause diseases. In order to avoid disease, a permanent lifestyle change is necessary. There are two types of fungal infections. Superficial infections can easily and quickly be remedied. These are conditions like ringworm, jock itch, and vaginal yeast infections. However, fungi can and do impregnate more deeply. These are called "deep mycoses." Depending on how long you have carried the fungus and how deeply it has penetrated, sometimes long-term therapy, including herbal remedies taken by mouth, and diet is necessary. In a 1992 research paper, Orian Truss, M. D., stated that sometimes a two to three year period of treatment is necessary to "clear" the body of fungal poisons.

We have confirmed his findings to be true in severe cases. In our experience, if a person had pesticide toxicity in his body or mercury toxicity (especially from mercury amalgam fillings in his teeth), he will clear fungi from his body slowly and be more prone to recurrence of fungi in the future.

Could the Initial Phase Diet be dangerous for anyone?
Since the IPD is high in proteins, people with advanced kidney disease should be very cautious while on the diet and should work closely with their physicians. In fact, someone with advanced kidney disease should probably avoid this diet since the kidneys may have a problem handling the protein load. The diet, however, will not cause kidney disease in one with healthy kidneys; in fact, it may even prevent kidney disease, according to numerous studies on atherosclerosis (a common cause of kidney damage).

Also, those who are pregnant or breast feeding or who are in childhood years may not be suited to this type of a diet due to the relative reduction of carbohydrates. Those who exercise vigorously may also not do well on a diet that restricts carbohydrates, as these can provide fuel for the body. If you fit into any of these categories, the diet should be discussed with us or your own nutritionist or doctor.

Why should I take psyllium hulls?

Psyllium, being a non-digestible fiber, is one of only three things known to bind fungal poisons (mycotoxins). The other two are charcoal and cholestyramine, a drug. (Costantini, A.V. *Fungalbionics: Cancer*. 1994.) Because psyllium is a fiber, it also regulates the bowels, relieving both constipation and diarrhea. It is imperative that as you kill fungus within the bowels, it is eliminated from the body.

People with gut problems, i.e., constipation, diarrhea, gas, bloating, reflux, etc., almost certainly have an "inflamed" or leaky gut. Psyllium hulls can greatly assist in sealing up the "leaky gut." Once the bowels are moving properly and the intestines are sealed, one can begin to absorb and assimilate nutrients from food. The use of organic foods is then recommended, since these are known to contain more nutrients.

Are psyllium hulls for everyone?

If you suffer from hypertension (high blood pressure), you may take psyllium, but do not take a brand of psyllium hulls that contains licorice, which can elevate blood pressure if taken regularly. Also, if you have any form of intestinal obstruction or have had surgery for intestinal obstruction, please get advice from a health professional prior to taking psyllium hulls.

What are fungi? How do they differ from bacteria?

Fungi are more highly developed than bacteria or viruses. They range from molds, mushrooms, and tiny round yeast spores to finger or string-like mycelial forms. The number of species of fungi is estimated to be in excess of one million. The number of fungal species implicated in human disease is around four hundred. Some fungi are *dimorphic*, or able to change forms. These can convert from natural, environmental mold forms to invasive round-cell tissue forms. A "*mycoses*" (pronounced 'my-ko-sees') describes a fungal infection of either the skin, deeper tissues, or organs within the human body. No tissue is immune to fungal proliferation.

Fungi (like humans) are heterotrophic, deriving nourishment from organic matter formed by other organisms. For fungi, this can be an animal that has died in the forest, leaves fallen from trees, or you and me! They thrive on warm, moist hosts. Fungi literally live everywhere: the soil, the air, in certain foods, even water. Many fungi are actually residents of the human body in healthy individuals (i.e., in the intestinal tract) and do not cause symptoms or diseases unless the person in which they are living becomes "immunocompromised." The opportunistic fungal organisms can then promote disease by either directly invading the tissues or by producing toxic by-products called *mycotoxins*. Mycotoxins can cause disease even in individuals who were initially healthy.

Bacteria, like fungi, are sometimes also normal residents of the human body. However, their physiology is quite different from fungi. This is why different drugs are used to kill bacteria than those used to kill fungi, though some drugs, sulfa drugs, for example, have both antibacterial and antifungal capabilities. There are harmless "good" bacteria and there are harmful "bad" bacteria. *Lactobacillus acidophilus* is one of several good bacteria that inhabit the small and large intestines and produce chemicals that inhibit the growth of bad bacteria and keep yeast and fungi counts under control. For example, *Lactobacillus acidophilus* produces chemicals that are toxic to the bacteria commonly known to cause "Montezuma's revenge." It is when these good bacteria succumb to antibiotics, chemicals in food, or chlorinated water that the normal balance is upset and the terrain of the bowel is changed. Without the protective bacteria, yeast can freely proliferate — this is when normal becomes abnormal and symptoms arise.

On your show, I hear you talk about fungi as the cause of many health problems. If this is true, why don't doctors know about this? -WM, Vancouver, Washington

You can imagine how many times we hear this question every day! We feel that the primary reason doctors don't understand the role of fungus in the disease process is lack of education. Not that your doctor is not educated, just the opposite is true. Fungal infections were very rare 50 years ago. In medicine, tradition is extremely valuable and breaking tradition does not often occur. Such is the case with fungal diseases.

Frankly, the reason that fungal infections were rare 50 years ago is because the pharmaceutical drugs that cause fungal infections were also rare or non-existent. To illustrate this point, in the April, 1996, issue of *Healthweek* magazine, writer Mary Ann Hellinghausen addressed the very question you have. The headline reads: **Fungal Infections Pose Dangers.** In this article, Dr. Michael G. Rinaldi says, "We can't neglect fungal diseases any longer." Dr. Rinaldi goes on to explain what we already know in our clinic: we just didn't see fungus infections 50 years ago. Why? Because we didn't have drugs that contributed to fungal growth! According to Dr. Rinaldi, "We're using antibiotics that are so powerful they save lives, but they also destroy normal flora, particularly in our intestinal tract. This allows pathogenic germs to colonize and eventually become infectious." Such is the case with fungal pathogens! It may take another decade, but more and more doctors are now recognizing not only the benefits but also the dangers inherent in prescriptive drugs.

I've heard that asthma can be caused by fungus. How do I tell if this is true in my case? -JM, Dallas, Texas

Do you remember when your asthma started? Was it following antibiotic, cortisone, or birth control pill usage? Although not exclusively due to these drugs, *bronchial pulmonary fungi* are sometimes misdiagnosed as asthma. A condition called farmer's lung may also appear to be asthma. With symptoms that are similar, even the brightest of asthma specialists miss fungus as the real root of some of these cases.

Systemic antifungal drugs that would get into the lungs and eradicate fungus can be tried. Ask your doctor about these.

I understand that fungi can spread from our intestines throughout the rest of the body. Can it also make it past the blood-brain barrier? -CM, Bangor, Maine

Yes, fungus can impregnate brain tissue, and such conditions are grave in that fungus can proliferate quickly and cause death. Since the inception of antibiotics, numerous publications have spoken about a condition called "meningeal fungi." In Chapter 5, we expound on this phenomenon of fungi within the tissues surrounding the brain possibly causing aberrant behavior. Dr. A. V. Costantini is publishing that hyperactivity may have its roots in mycotoxins (fungal poisons). If this is the case, it is highly likely that other brain malfunctions may also be due to fungi.

How does fungus get into our bodies? Do we eat it?
-BB, Portland, Oregon

Let's answer your second question, first. In a book called *Industrial Microbiology* there is a list of foods that ferment. The fermentation of foods takes place in the presence of fungi. For

253

example, the fungus *Rhizopus* ferments soybeans into tempeh. Soybean is a relatively common food in the American diet. Then one must consider the food chain when concerning ourselves with fungi in our diet. The fungal poison aflatoxin B1 is one of the most deadly poisons known to exist. Corn, stored in warm, moist, mildewing silos, can become impregnated with the deadly mold that produces this mycotoxin. Government regulations prohibit human consumption of corn infested with detectable levels of aflatoxin B1 (20 parts per billion), but they don't prohibit animals from consuming it! Corn infested with 300 parts per billion is fed to chickens and cattle. And who eats the chickens and cattle? You get the picture!

Another way fungus enters our systems is through contact with the soil. For those of you who like to garden, a cut or abrasion on the skin opens a passageway for soil-based fungi. Let's not forget that once fungi have gained access to our bodies, drugs like antibiotics, cortisone, and birth control pills can either initiate or exacerbate fungal proliferation. This is sometimes dangerous, given that their fuel is the standard American diet — SAD! — a diet often loaded with an extraordinary amount of sugar.

Your Fungal Quotient
A Symptom Questionnaire

*Assessing the odds that microscopic fungi
lie behind a given condition*

The following questionnaire is designed to aid you in measuring how much you have been exposed to fungi and their mycotoxins. Physicians may also use this questionnaire to assess their patients' histories.

Because the degree of exposure varies from incident to incident, and because consumption of natural, antifungal nutrients can often neutralize a portion of such exposure, we are unable to provide a meaningful index to which you might map your final score. However, a high number of positive answers would suggest that your condition has been caused by fungi and their mycotoxins. If a couple of weeks on the Antifungal Program improves your health, very likely a fungus does lie at the root of your problem.

Fungal Quotient Questionnaire

1. Have you ever taken repeated or prolonged rounds of antibiotics? If so, how long ago, and for what conditions?

2. Have you taken repeated or prolonged courses of steroids or cortisone-based pills? If so, how long ago, and for what reason?

3. Have you been diagnosed with fibromyalgia?

4. Do you have, or have you ever had asthma?

5. Have you been diagnosed with arthritis?

6. Do you have diabetes? Type 1 or type 2?

7. At any time in your life, have you been treated for worms or other parasites?

8. Have you traveled to less developed countries? When and where?

9. Have you ever been diagnosed with cancer? If so, were you treated with chemotherapy or radiation?

10. Do you have, or have you had, ringworm, fingernail or toenail fungus, or jock itch?

11. Have you ever been diagnosed with attention-deficit disorder?
a. If so, are you currently taking medications for your condition?
b. Name the medication(s).

12. If you are currently ill, were you in and around areas such as construction sites at the time you became sick?

13. Do you suffer from fatigue? Based on a 1-10 scale, with 10 representing the worst, how bad has your fatigue been the past few weeks?

14. Do you suffer from irritability, frequent memory loss, or a feeling of constantly being "spaced out?"

15. Do your muscles, bones, or joints bother you? Would you describe them as aching, weak, stiff, or swollen?

16. Do you get headaches?
a. How long have you suffered with headaches?
b. How many days per month do you have headaches?
c. Do you think your headaches may be hormonally driven?
d. What medication do you take for these headaches?

17. Do you have itching, tingling, or burning skin?

18. Do you have hives, psoriasis, dandruff, or chronic skin rashes?

19. Do you have acne?

20. Are you on medications for the skin problems listed in questions 17, 18 and 19? Name the medication(s).

21. Have you experienced hair loss, itching in your inner ear, or vision problems?

22. Do you have high blood pressure, low blood pressure, high cholesterol or triglycerides? If so, are you on medications for these problems? How long have you taken these medications?

23. Do you have mitral valve prolapse or heart symptoms, i.e., racing pulse or uncontrolled heart beat? If so, are you on medications for this condition? How long have you taken these medications?

24. Have you ever been diagnosed with an autoimmune disease?

25. Are you bothered by recurrent digestive problems, including bloating, belching, gas, constipation, diarrhea, abdominal pain, indigestion, or reflux? If so, are you on medication for these problems? How long have you been taking these medications?

26. Do you have chronic infections for which your doctor keeps prescribing antibiotics? If so, what are these infections, and how long have they been recurring?

27. Does your condition worsen in response to the heat from taking a shower or a bath? Does very hot weather make it worse?

28. Do your symptoms worsen on damp days or in musty, moldy environments?

29. On days when the mold/pollen count is elevated, do you feel worse?

30. Do you often feel "blue" or depressed?
a. Are you presently seeing a therapist for depression?
b. Are you on medication for depression?
c. If so, how long have you taken these medications?

31. Do you drink alcohol? If so, how often, how much, and for how long have you been doing so?

32. Do you smoke? If so, how often, how much, and for how many years have you been smoking?

33. Do you often crave sugar?

34. Do you tend to eat a lot of corn and peanuts?

35. Have you ever spent a lot of time on a farm?

36. Have you experienced mold-related problems in your home or office? Has your home or office ever flooded?

37. Are you allergic to pollens, molds, animal dander, dust, mites, perfumes, chemicals, smoke, or fabric store odors? Do you presently take allergy shots?

38. Are you allergic to any foods? Have you had food allergy tests run? Were these skin tests or blood tests?

For Women Only

39. Have you ever taken birth control pills? If so, have you ever experienced complications as a result? Please describe you reaction.

40. Have you ever been bothered by vaginal or urinary tract problems?

41. Are your ovaries, thyroid gland, adrenals, and pancreas functioning as they should? Have you experienced symptoms possibly indicating hormonal disturbances, such as PMS, menstrual irregularities, loss of libido, infertility, sugar cravings, weight problems, or feeling inappropriately hot or cold? If so, are you on medications for these problems? How long have you taken these medications?

For Men Only

41. Have you ever felt pain in your testicles unrelated to injury?

42. Have you ever been bothered with prostate problems?

43. Are your testicles, thryoid gland, adrenals, and pancreas functioning as they should? Have you experienced symptoms that possibly indicate hormonal disturbances, such as loss of libido, infertility, impotence, sugar cravings, weight problems, and constantly feeling hot or cold? If so, are you on medications for any of these conditions? How long have you taken these medications?

A high yes/no ratio may mean that the degree to which you are exposed to fungi puts you at risk for disease. If you suspect you are at risk, or that you may have already contracted a fungal infection, you should consider making some immediate changes to your life-style. Try the Initial Phase Diet, exercise under supervision of a physician, and get on some strong, natural or prescriptive, antifungal medications for a time. Once again, please do so under the supervision of your doctor. If you health improves, or if it worsens for period of a few days or weeks before returning to normal, quite likely a fungus lay at the root of your problem. Keep a close watch on your symptoms, returning to the Initial Phase diet from time to time, as necessary.

A Week of the Initial Phase Diet
Example menus

We've gotten a lot of questions as to what a menu based on the Initial Phase diet would look like. The layout below is not meant to be followed verbatim. And, *Initial Phase* almost always requires more than a week to achieve results. Note the emphasis on water, and refer to our recipe section/website for details on certain dishes.

Monday
Breakfast:	Fried eggs, uncured bacon, ½ grapefruit
Snack:	Almonds, water (always bottled or filtered)
Lunch:	Tuna with celery. Herbal tea
Snack:	Carrot sticks, water
Dinner:	Steak, steamed veggies, sparkling lime water
Dessert: (optional)	Plain yogurt with raspberries

Tuesday
Breakfast:	Omelet with onions, leeks, parsley, and chopped bacon
Snack:	Celery sticks, water
Lunch:	Chicken salad with *Initial Phase Diet* dressing
Snack:	Cashews, water
Dinner:	Salmon fillets with lemon and butter, avocado salad
Dessert: (optional)	Green apple

Wednesday
Breakfast:	Poached eggs, freshly squeezed carrot juice
Snack:	Walnuts, water
Lunch:	Broccoli chicken without rice, herbal tea
Snack:	Grapefruit, water
Dinner:	Steak, spinach salad with lemon juice and olive oil dressing
Dessert: (optional)	Plain yogurt with chopped pecans and fresh cranberries

Thursday

Breakfast: Scrambled eggs with breakfast steak

Snack: Green apple wedges, almonds, herbal tea

Lunch: Tuna salad with lettuce

Snack: Broccoli, cauliflower, water

Dinner: Halibut with sautéed vegetables

Dessert: Yogurt with fresh blueberries
(optional)

Friday

Breakfast: Freshly squeezed carrot juice, hard boiled eggs

Snack: Celery sticks or green apple wedges with almond butter

Lunch: Beef patties, steamed and buttered asparagus

Snack: Sunflower seeds, water

Dinner: Kaufmann's favorite meal (see recipes)

Dessert: ½ grapefruit
(optional)

Saturday

Breakfast: Omelet with green onions, bacon, spinach leaves

Snack: Carrot sticks

Lunch: Cucumber salad w/ onions, tomatoes, black olives, olive oil

Snack: Pecans, yogurt with blackberries, water

Dinner: Steak with steamed broccoli

Dessert: Sautéed green apples and cranberries with roasted pecans
(optional) and whipping cream

Sunday

Breakfast: Freshly squeezed carrot juice, ½ grapefruit, poached eggs

Snack: Pumpkin seeds, water

Lunch: Salad with grilled tuna, herbal tea

Snack: Celery sticks, water

Dinner: Stir-fried chicken, broccoli, snow peas, squash with butter

Dessert: Almonds, chamomile tea
(optional)

Recipes

for the Initial Phase and InterPhase diets

Kaufmann's Favorite Meal

Dice: tomatoes, onions, cucumbers, avocado, and black olives.
Add: hard-boiled eggs and either smoked salmon or cubes of beef purchased from a health food market.
Toss: Add two tablespoons of olive or grape seed oil and the juice from a fresh-squeezed lemon as the dressing.

Spinach Salad

1 bunch spinach, torn or sliced to desired size	1 cucumber, sliced
1/2 to 1 cup cauliflowerettes	6 radishes, sliced (opt.)
1 - 2 stalks celery, chopped	2 eggs, hard-boiled & sliced

Toss together all ingredients. Flavor as desired with herbs and spices. Serve with lemon and oil dressing.

Nine Vegetable Cocktail

1 pint fresh tomatoes	1 green pepper, sliced
1 cucumber, sliced	1 lettuce leaf
1 radish, quartered	a few sprigs parsley
1/4 onion, sliced	1 stalk celery
1 slender carrot	1 pint ice cubes, to desired consistency

In an electric blender, blend together all ingredients, adding ice cubes a few at a time. If juice freezes, blend a little longer before adding remaining ice. Add salt and pepper or other herbs and spices to taste. Increase ice for colder or thinner juice. Makes 1-1/2 quarts.

Almost Tartar Sauce

1/2 cup green onions, tops included, coarsely chopped

1 tsp. sea salt

1/4 tsp. pepper

1/4 to 1/2 tsp. Mrs. Dash

1/4 cup parsely, no heavy stems, coarsely chopped

1/4 cup cucumber, finely chopped

juice of 1/2 to 1 freshly squeezed lemon

1 tsp. capers

1 pint plain yogurt

Combine all ingredients except yogurt in a bowl, tossing to blend. Feed mixture through a meat grinder using the coarse blade, or use a blender on 'chop.' Stir results into yogurt. Chill.

Serve with fish, or with slices, chunks, or cubes of any vegetable.

Basic Vege-yogurt Dip

1/2 c. plain yogurt

sea salt to taste

spices and herbs as desired

juice of 1/2 lemon

Spices and herbs might include garlic, chives, marjoram, or thyme. Mix together all ingredients. Chill and serve.

Herb Dressing

1 tsp. dry mustard

1 tbsp. fresh parsley, chopped

1 tsp. dill weed

1/4 tsp. freshly ground, black pepper

pinch thyme

1/2 cup virgin olive oil

Stir together all ingredients except olive oil until dry mustard is dissolved. Allow to sit for ten minutes. Blend in olive oil, beginning with 1/3 cup and adding additional oil to taste.

Use to dress green salads or serve with slices, chunks, or cubes of any vegetable.

Mexican Relish

1 lb. tomatillos, peeled	1 clove garlic
2 pinches cumin	2 serrano chilis
1/2 onion, minced	1/2 tbsp. butter

Blend together all ingredients. Melt butter in a skillet. Sautee mixture until onions and tomatillos are clear. Serve with chicken, fish, or other vegetables. Store leftover relish in the refrigerator.

Salad Dressing and Vegetable Marinade

1/2 cup olive oil	1 tsp. oregano
juice of 2 lemons	1 tsp. garlic powder

Mix together all ingredients in a pint jar. Fill jar the rest of the way with water. Shake well to mix, then pour over whole, sliced, chunked or chopped vegetables. Squash, radishes, cucumbers, broccoli, carrots, bell pepper, cauliflower, and onions work well. Refrigerate, allowing to marinate two hours or longer. Add other herbs and spices to taste.

To use over spinach or lettuce, add just prior to serving.

Curried Cauliflower

1 - 2 cups cauliflowerettes

1 onion, thinly sliced

1/2 cup fat-skimmed chicken stock

1/2 tsp. butter

1 tsp. curry powder, or to taste

1/2 tsp. cumin (opt.)

Combine ingredients in a small pan, cover. Simmer until most of the liquid has evaporated.

Variation: Other vegetables may be "curried" in this manner.

Deviled Eggs

6 hard boiled eggs, halved lengthwise

paprika to taste

2 tsp. dry mustard

2 Tbsp. plain yogurt

salt and pepper to taste

Separate yolks from whites. Mash yolks together in a small bowl. Add remaining ingredients, mixing well. Refill egg whites with yolk mixture. Arrange on a platter and sprinkle with additional paprika.

Beef Patties

1 lb. ground beef

1/2 tsp. sea salt

1/8 tsp. garlic powder

1 cup onion, finely chopped or 2 tsp. dried onion

1/4 tsp. black pepper

Mix together all ingredients. Shape into six patties. Broil or grill to desired doneness. Ground chicken, turkey or lamb may be used in place of beef. If lamb is used, add a pinch of oregano.

Chicken Stroganoff

1 lb. chicken, chopped or ground	1 tsp. sea salt
	1/4 tsp. pepper
1 med. onion, chopped	1/2 tsp. thyme
1 clove garlic, minced	fresh parsley, chopped
1 cup chicken broth	2 Tbsp. olive oil

Heat oil in a wide frying pan over medium to high heat. Lightly brown the chicken. Just as chicken begins to brown, add onion and garlic, stirring until onion becomes limp and translucent. Add broth, salt, pepper, and thyme. Simmer, stirring frequently until thickened. Serve with brown rice. Garnish with fresh parsley.

Fish Fillet Almondine

2 lbs. fish fillets (snapper, cod, sole)	1 Tbsp. lemon juice
1/4 c. olive oil or butter	1/2 tsp. garlic salt
3 Tbsp. slivered almonds	1/4 tsp. pepper

Heat 2 Tbsp. oil in large skillet. Add almonds and sautee 2 to 3 minutes, stirring constantly until golden brown. Remove almonds and set aside. In remaining oil, cook fish 3 to 4 minutes on each side until fish flakes when pierced with fork. Transfer to warm platter. Add lemon juice, salt, pepper and almonds to pan drippings; spoon over fish.

Lemon-Fried Chicken

1 fryer chicken, skin removed	1/4 tsp. marjoram
	1/8 tsp. pepper
1/4 c. fresh lemon juice	1/2 tsp. grated lemon rind
1/4 tsp. garlic salt	2 Tbsp. butter
3/4 tsp. sea salt	1/4 tsp. thyme

Cut chicken into pieces and place in a large, shallow pan. Mix together the remaining ingredients, except the butter. Pour mixture over chicken and marinate in the refrigerator for at least three hours, turning occasionally. Drain chicken on absorbent paper.

Preheat skillet, and add butter. Add chicken and cook for 15 minutes with lid partially on. Turn chicken and continue cooking for 10 minutes with lid partially on. Place cover on tightly and cook for 15 minutes more.

Mexican Fish

1 - 2 lbs. fish, whole or fillets	1 lb. peeled tomatillos (Mexican green tomatoes)
1 clove garlic, freshly chopped	2 pinches cumin
1 lime, freshly juiced	1 clove garlic
pepper to taste, white or black	1/2 onion, minced
1 small onion, chopped	2 serrano chilis (opt.)

Pierce fish on each side with fork. Rub garlic into fish, pour fresh lime juice on inside and outside of fish, then sprinkle with pepper.

Marinate two hours. Place, with chopped onion, in cold skillet that maintains an even temperature. Leave on medium heat eight minutes, turn fish over, and cook until done, approximately ten minutes more.

Blend together remaining ingredients. Heat in separate skillet until onion and tomatillos are clear. Pour onto warm platter and top with cooked fish.

Note: this recipe contains no salt. The garlic and lime make it unnecessary.

Old Fashioned Pot Roast

3 lb. lean brisket of beef	1 large onion, chopped
1 clove garlic, minced	1 small bay leaf
	1/2 tsp. sea salt
1/2 tsp. black pepper, coarsely ground	a variety of vegetables, cut into pieces

Preheat oven to 450 degrees. Rub meat with garlic and pepper; place in a greased Dutch oven or heavy saucepan. Brown for 10 minutes on each side.

Slowly and carefully add 1 cup water and remaining ingredients. May also add cleaned, cut vegetables such as carrots, celery, bell peppers, or rutabaga for a simple, one dish meal.

Reduce oven temperature to 300 degrees. Cover and bake 3 hours or until tender.

Makes approximately 10 servings.

271

Turkey Salad

1 cup turkey, cooked and diced

2 cup rice, chilled

1 cup celery, diced

1 medium-sized, green pepper, shredded

2 Tbsp. parsley, chopped

1/2 c. olive oil

1/3 c. lemon juice

1/2 tsp. curry

1 Tbsp. pimento, chopped

Mix together turkey, rice, and vegetables; chill. Combine oil, lemon juice, and curry; let stand for 1 hour. Pour dressing over salad just before serving.

Tuna Salad

1/2 c. plain yogurt

1 Tbsp. lemon juice

1/4 tsp. sea salt or Mrs. Dash

1 jalapeno pepper, chopped (optional!)

1 12-oz. can tuna, crumbled

1 small onion, sliced

1 stalk celery, coarsely chopped

Lightly blend all ingredients. Chill and serve with slices, chunks, or cubes of any vegetable.

Makes approximately 1-1/2 cups.

Index

About **Doug Kaufmann**

Doug Kaufmann is a nationally recognized author, lecturer, television and radio show host, with more than 30 years of experience in diversified health care.

Kaufmann served as a Navy hospital corpsman in Vietnam, where he was honored with the Combat Action Ribbon, Vietnamese Cross of Gallantry and the Vietnam Service Medal, one bronze star.

After Vietnam, Kaufmann added an American Society of Allergy Technicians certification to his Navy training. While working in allergy/immunology with a Los Angeles specialist, he studied food allergies at the Washington University School of Medicine. He co-investigated several research papers with doctors at USC Medical School. Later, he opened a laboratory and staffed it with four, research immunologists focused on food and fungal research. The lab devised the first ELISA tests for food allergy, and it conducted significant research aimed at better understanding the food-disease link.

A group of Texas physicians recruited Kaufmann in 1987. During subsequent research in Dallas, he saw many patients with various, apparently incurable diseases responded favorably to dietary changes and antifungal drugs.

Kaufmann began broadcasting his findings in nutrition on Texas radio in 1992. His "At A Glance" vignettes continue to be broadcast daily by more than 200 radio stations. He transitioned to television in 1999, as host of the nationally broadcast program, *Your Health*. The show empowers its viewers to take possession of their own health. *Your Health* is currently broadcast in more than 160 cities throughout the United States.

Kaufmann's other books include *The Food Sensitivity Diet* (1984), *The Germ That Causes Cancer* (2002), and *Infectious Diabetes* (2003). Each book offers an alternative viewpoint to prevailing medical thought on the diagnosis and treatment of disease.

Currently, Kaufmann and Dr. Holland devote most of their time to research and writing, and holding seminars on their findings throughout the United States.

Kaufmann and his wife, Ruth, have been married for more than 20 years. They live with their two sons in a Dallas suburb.

About **Dr. David Holland, M.D.**

David Holland is the Medical Communications Director at MediaTrition, Inc. He works documenting the roles fungi and fungal toxins play in common, human illnesses, and communicating his findings to the medical community.

Dr. Holland holds a B.S. in Microbiology from Texas Tech University. Since obtaining his M.D. from Texas Tech University Health Sciences Center in 1993, he has worked in primary care, urgent care, occupational and nutritional medicine. He is a Diplomat of the American Board of Family Practice, as well as the American Board of Ambulatory Medicine.

Dr. Holland joined Doug Kaufmann in operating a nutritional medicine clinic in Dallas, Texas in 1996. He went on to complete his residency at John Peter Smith Hospital in Ft. Worth, Texas in 2002, and is currently Board Certified in Family Practice.

Dr. Holland is married with two children. He stays in shape by jogging and running in the occasional marathon.

Patrick Kwan, MSc. received his BSc. in Microbiology from the University of California, Riverside. He graduated with an MSc. from Oregon State University. Mr. Kwan is a founding member of Diversified Research, the largest food laboratory in Canada. For 13 years, he was a senior consultant to George Weston, Ltd., the largest retail food chain in Canada.

Milt Gearing, Ph.D. received his doctorate in clinical psychology from the University of South Carolina. Dr. Gearing was formerly director of Psychological Services, Charter Hospital, Dallas.

Nathan L. Lipton, M.D. is a Fellow of the American Academy of Ophthalmologists, and Diplomate of the American Board of Ophthalmology.

C. R. Mabray, M.D. is a Fellow of the American College of Obstetricians and Gynecologists.

Richard Becker, D.O. has spent 15 years in family practice. He received his B.A. in biochemistry from Loma Linda University, a world leader in nutritional therapies, and his graduate degree from the Health Science College of Osteopathic Medicine, Kansas City, Missouri. Dr. Becker is a Hodgkins lymphoma survivor. He follows Doug Kaufmann's nutritional approach to the treatment of cancer.